NYMPHS AND NAIADS

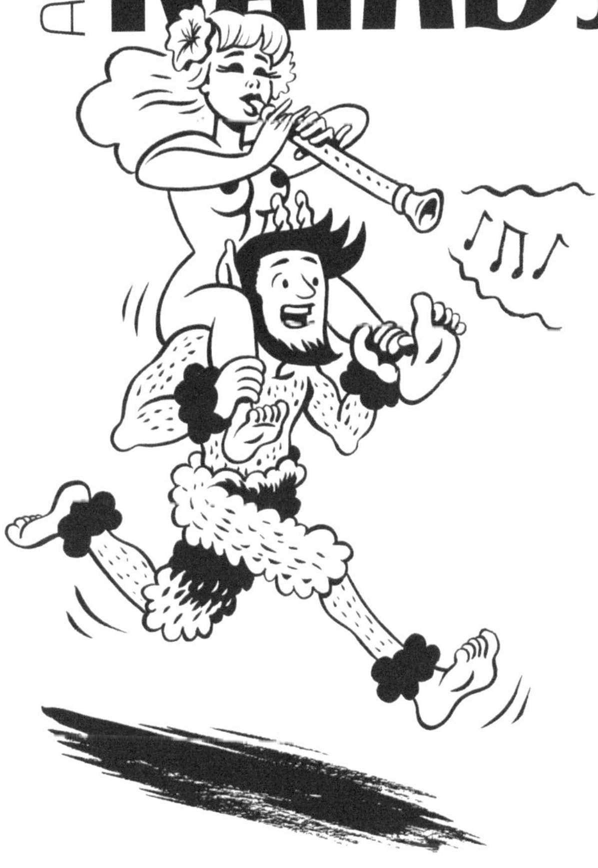

Published in 2021 by Wolfbait Books © 2021

www.wolfbait.co.uk

ISBN: 978-1-9162151-6-0

A catalogue record of this book is available at the British Library.

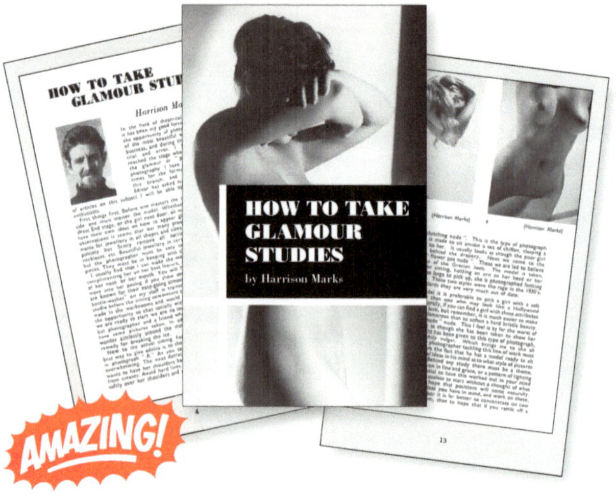

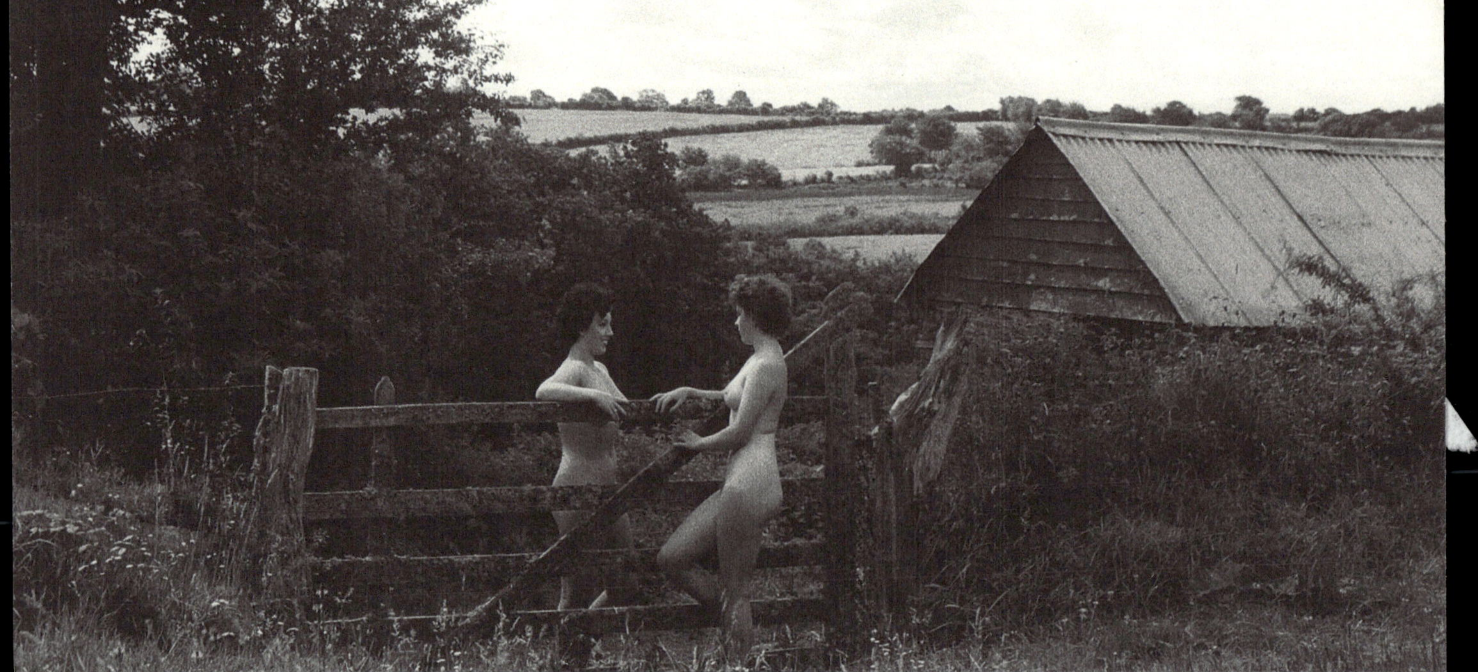

NYMPHS AND NAIADS

By Yahya El-Droubie

Photography by Stephen Glass

Illustrations by Colin Gordon

WOLFBAIT
UNDER THE COUNTER CULTURE

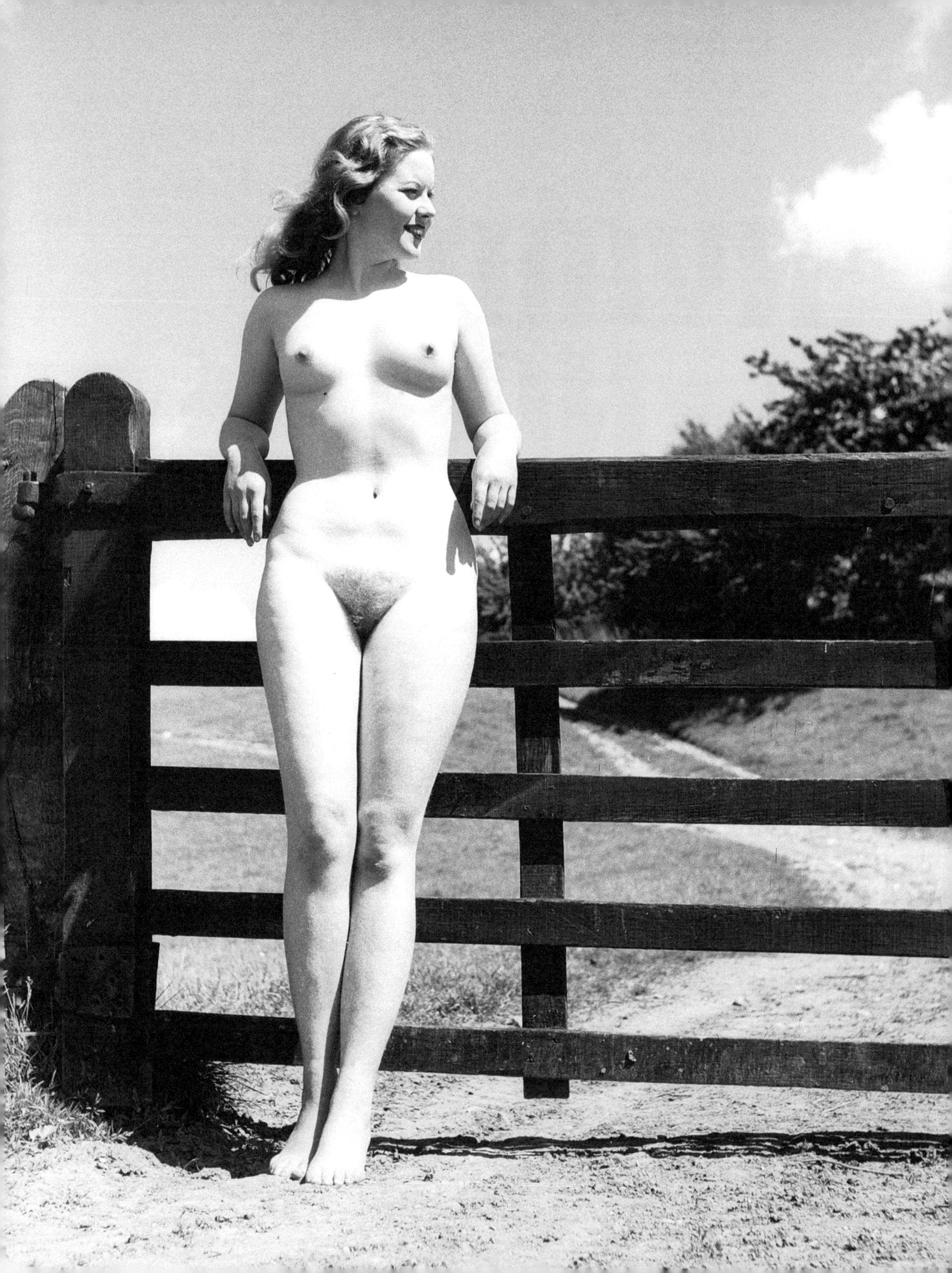

Introduction

THE PHOTOGRAPHER STEPHEN GLASS is something of an enigma. He was sufficiently well known during the 1950s for his name to be prominently displayed on magazine covers to help sell them, but very little was written about him or his work at that time. The opposite is true of his elder brother, Zoltán, who was also a photographer. Known to his friends as "Zolly", Zoltán was featured and interviewed in numerous magazines on both sides of the Atlantic.

And ne'er did Grecian chisel trace,
a Nymph, a Naiad or a Grace,
Of finer form, or lovelier face!

— Sir Walter Scott,
The Lady of the Lake, 1810.

Zoltán Glass was born in Budapest, Hungary, on April 26, 1903. He began his career as a cartoonist and retoucher for a local newspaper, but in 1925 he moved to Berlin, where he was employed as the picture editor of an evening newspaper; he then moved on to the *Berliner Tagblatt* as a photojournalist. Zoltán prospered and was soon able to develop a thriving freelance business as a commercial photographer and journalist. He established Reclaphot, a photographic agency that specialised in advertising work, and Autophot, a company dedicated exclusively to automobile photography. A keen motor sport enthusiast and amateur racer, Zoltán covered Germany's biggest races at the Nürburgring and Avus circuits. His most famous photographs are of the Mercedes-Benz Silver Arrows team, which dominated Grand Prix racing in the mid-1930s.

With the rise of Hitler, business became increasingly difficult in Germany, and Zoltán fled to London. As an enemy alien at the outbreak of World War II, he was not permitted to pursue his profession and faced the threat of internment, so he voluntarily handed over his camera equipment to the British authorities.

After the war, Zoltán eked out a living taking publicity stills for clients in the film and theatre worlds. His career took a big step up when fellow Hungarian Arpad Elfer, Creative Director of Colman, Prentis & Varley, one of the most prestigious London ad agencies, started giving him work. By the mid-1950s, he was one of the most successful fashion and advertising photographers in the capital, with a studio at 183 Kings Road, Chelsea, and later another at 41 Paradise Walk, SW3.

Left: Claudia Gray.

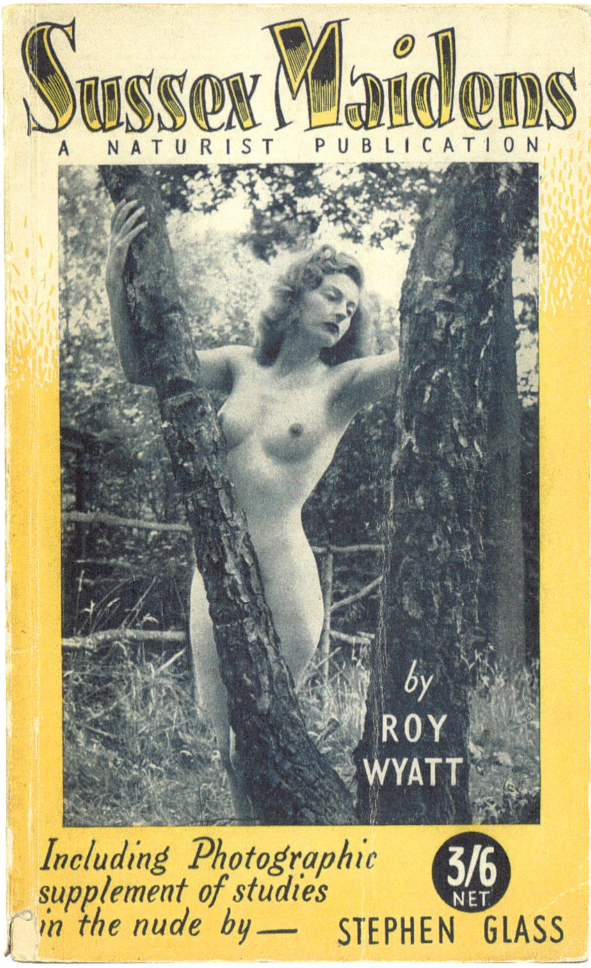

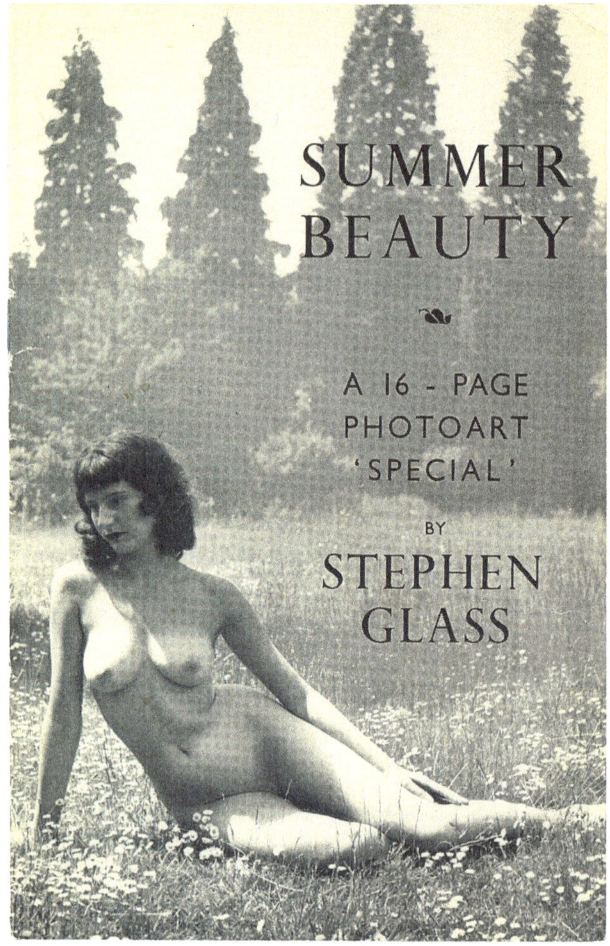

One of his clients was Odhams Press, who published *Lilliput*, a pocket-sized gentleman's magazine that featured an assortment of titillating articles and risqué humour, together with adventurous photographic essays from such well-known talents as Bill Brandt and Brassai.

Zoltán's brother, Stephen, who also fled Europe during World War II, carved out a name for himself taking pictures for such publications as *The Naturist* and *Health and Efficiency.* The well-known model Pamela Green (1929–2010) posed for him several times at the infamous nudist camp Spielplatz in Bricket Wood, Hertfordshire, and at his tiny first-floor studio in Old Church Street, just off the Kings Road in Chelsea. *"In those days, when Stephen photographed me, I still had dark hair. He liked his props, especially stuffed animals,"* she said. Pamela's agent,

Above left: *Sussex Maidens* by Roy Wyatt, published by The Naturist Ltd., 1949. Cover model Adrienne Germaine.

Above right: *Summer Beauty,* a 16-page photoart special by Stephen Glass. c.1952.

Right: Claudia Gray.

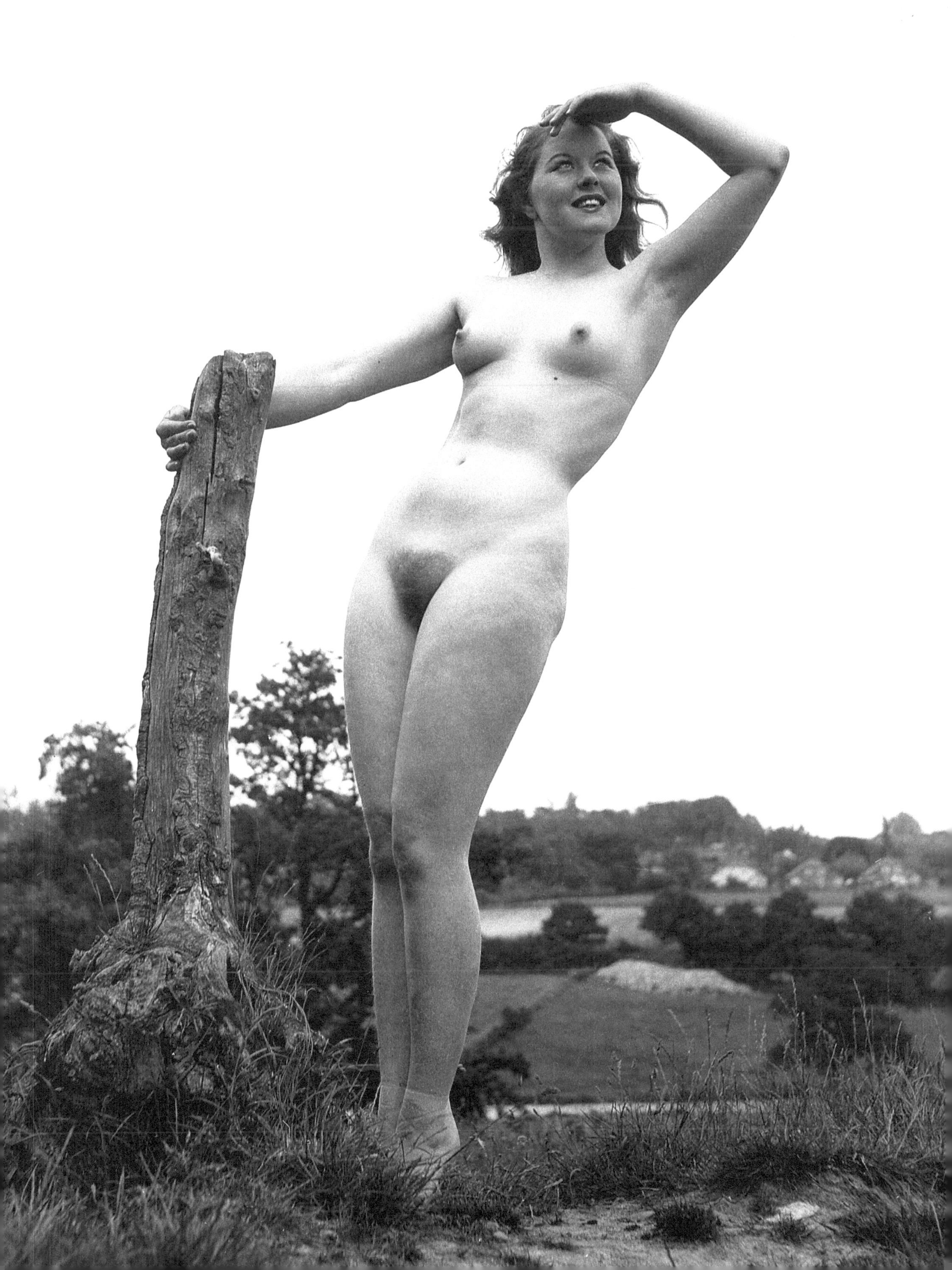

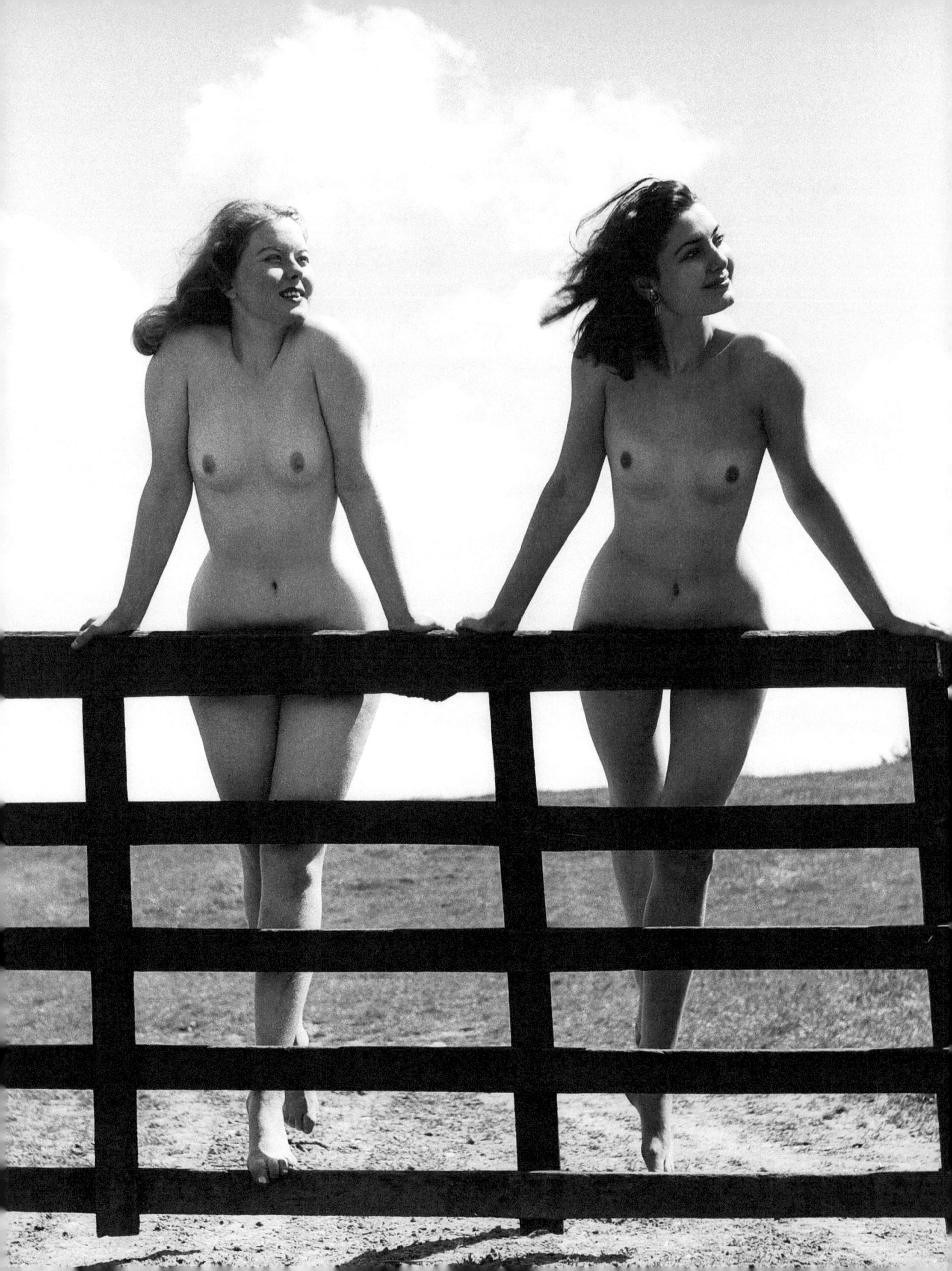

Pearl Beresford, sent her along to Zoltán, whose studio on the Kings Road was enormous by comparison. Unlike Stephen, Zoltán was brisk and businesslike.

Iseult, the daughter of Spielplatz co-founders Charles and Dorothy Macaskie, remembers Stephen. *"He would often ask me to pose for him,"* she said. *"I quite enjoyed having my photo taken, but when I asked to be paid, he stop using me. A bit of pocket money back then would have been nice."*

As well as magazines, Stephen's work graced a series of small books published by The Naturist Ltd., such as *Sussex Maidens* (1949), *The Pool of Enchantment* (1950) and *Nudist Life in Spielplatz* (1956). He also photographed the popular model June Palmer (1940–2004). The photos in this book are from his uncensored negatives. Until the end of the 1960s, it was considered obscene to show pubic hair or genitalia in British publications. To ensure that an image of a naked young lady would not incur the wrath of the censor, the model would shave down below and the photograph would then be retouched by hand to erase anything problematic.

By 1964, Zoltán Glass had made enough money to sell his Chelsea studios to a consortium of British photographers. He then moved to a villa in Roquebrune on the French Riviera with his common-law wife Pat, a former cabaret dancer. He offered his collection of pin-up photography to glamour photographer Harrison Marks who, strangely, turned it down. Zoltán died in France on February 24, 1981, at the age of 78, leaving neither offspring nor a will. His photographs were eventually given to The National Science and Media Museum in Bradford, Yorkshire. Stephen Glass died on 23 April, 1990. His work ended up at auction.

In my Pantheon, Pan still reigns in his pristine glory, with his ruddy face, his flowing beard, and his shaggy body, his pipe and his crook, his nymph Echo, and his chosen daughter Iambe; for the great god Pan is not dead, as was rumoured. No god ever dies. Perhaps of all the gods of New England and of ancient Greece, I am most constant at his shrine.

— Henry David Thoreau

Left: Claudia Gray and Rita Wheatley.

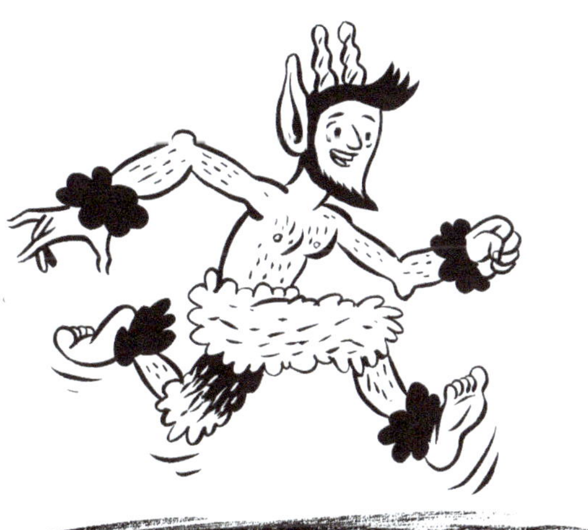

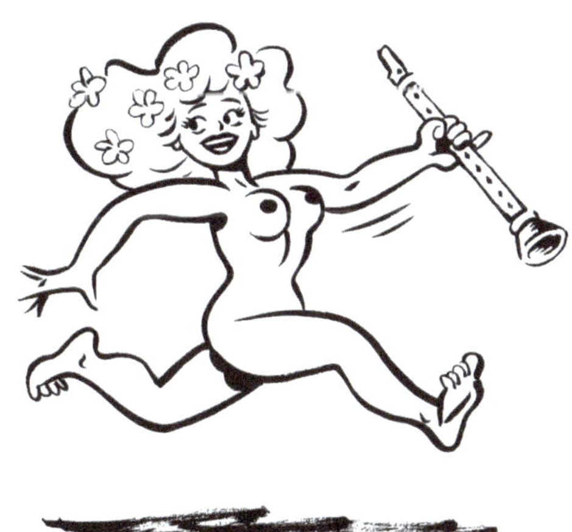

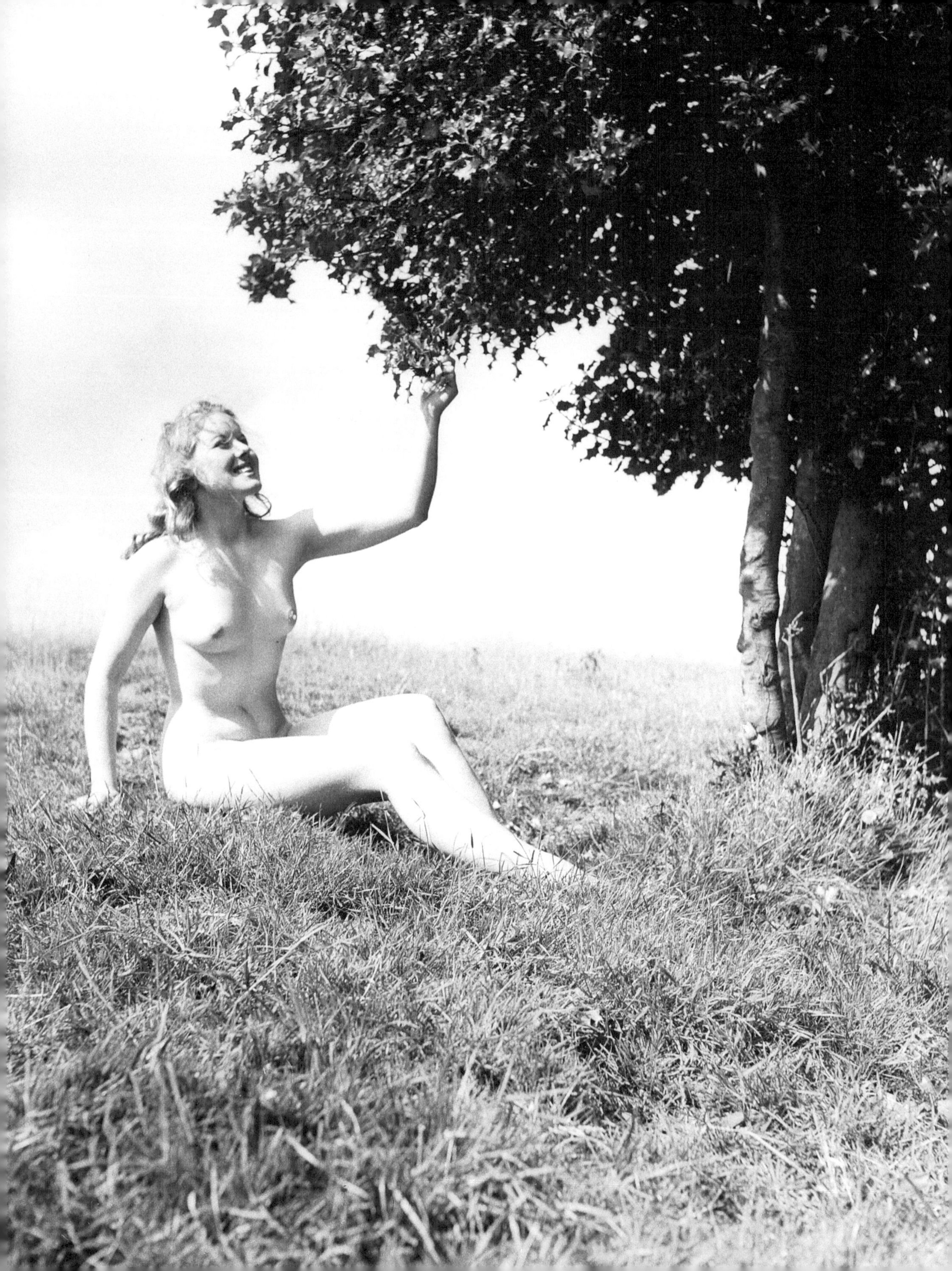

Due, in part, to the censorship laws of the 1950s, photographers often sought to cloak their work in respectability, using Classical allusions in an attempt to validate their "art studies". There is a certain naive charm to captioning a photograph of a lady in a state of undress *Nymph in a Sunlit Glade* or *Nymph Surprised*, and we shouldn't underestimate the hunger for art from the boys behind the bike shed or the homesick squaddie in barracks. Be that as it may, there's also something much deeper at play.

At the end of the 19th century, several groups embraced a broad philosophy whose central belief was that nudity is a natural state that should be widely adopted for the betterment of society. This philosophy was associated with an idealisation of ancient Greek mythology and a reimagining of Arcadia, the unspoiled wilderness homeland of the god Pan and assorted non-human creatures. Along with Pan, female divinities called nymphs, who presided over natural features such as trees, mountains and water, became all the rage.

No doubt this was part of the wider zeitgeist; after all, Arcadia, along with Pan, was a common subject in the work of late Victorian and Edwardian painters and authors. In literature, Pan can be found in poetry, novels and even children's books. Pan, a phallic deity widely associated with lustful and rampant sexuality, was reinvented as a benevolent, genial god of woodland and meadow — a symbol of a lost pastoral world. He appears in this benign and gentler form in Kenneth Graham's 1908 novel *The Wind in the Willows*, in the somewhat surprising chapter called "The Piper at the Gates of Dawn", from which Pink Floyd's debut studio album takes its name.*

Was this Edwardian cult of Pan a response to the industrialisation and destruction of nature and the old rural ways at the end of the 19th century? A destruction which broke the last vestiges of meaningful connection between the vast majority of urbanised Britons and the English countryside. Who knows, but from around 1890 the cult of Pan grew deep roots within the popular consciousness of the British public.

Even though the age of Pisces was making way for the Age of Aquarius, the cult of Pan came to an abrupt end with the First World War. In the novel *Blessing of Pan* (1927) by Lord Dunsany, the nuanced treatment of the themes of paganism, nature worship, and anti-industrialisation seem like an elegy.

When men begin to think that the Golden Age belongs solely to ancient history, that the future holds no radiant beauty, no effulgence of glory for the human race, mankind will be in a state of dotage. We nudists know the joy of conviction that the best is yet to be.

— *American Sunbather,* 1960

Left: Claudia Grey.

* On Guy Fawkes night in 1966 Pink Floyd played a gig at Fiveacres nudist club.

Right: *Sussex Maidens*, "The Girl on the Farm", 1949, page 23. Orginal caption: Sussex has been an agricultural county for as long as anyone can remember, but this young lady is content to pose in front of the haystack and leave the farm work to someone else.

But the pagan gods were just reinventing themselves for the new age. The English Gymnosophical Society was formed in 1922 and became the New Gymnosophy Society in 1926 — the word gymnosophy comes from the Greek words naked and wisdom. The society helped fund the purchase of land at Bricket Wood in Hertfordshire for what was to become Britain's first nudist club site; it was named Fouracres. After the Second World War, it evolved into the Fiveacres Country Club and with the involvement of Gerald Gardner, "the father of witchcraft", became a front for Wiccans, as witchcraft was illegal in England until 1951.

In 1933 Margaret Murray wrote of Pan in her book *The God of the Witches*, in which she theorised that Pan was one form of the ancient Horned God who was worshipped by the Witch Cult throughout Europe.

So it's clear that the Edwardian cult of Pan, Wicca, neopaganism, and the nudist movement have intertwined roots. And therefore a picture of a naked young lady standing in a clearing in the woods captioned *Nymph in a Sunlit Glade* is not just a cynical ploy for approval or ironic kitsch, but part of a long history of folkloric and counter-culture visions of a very British Arcadia.

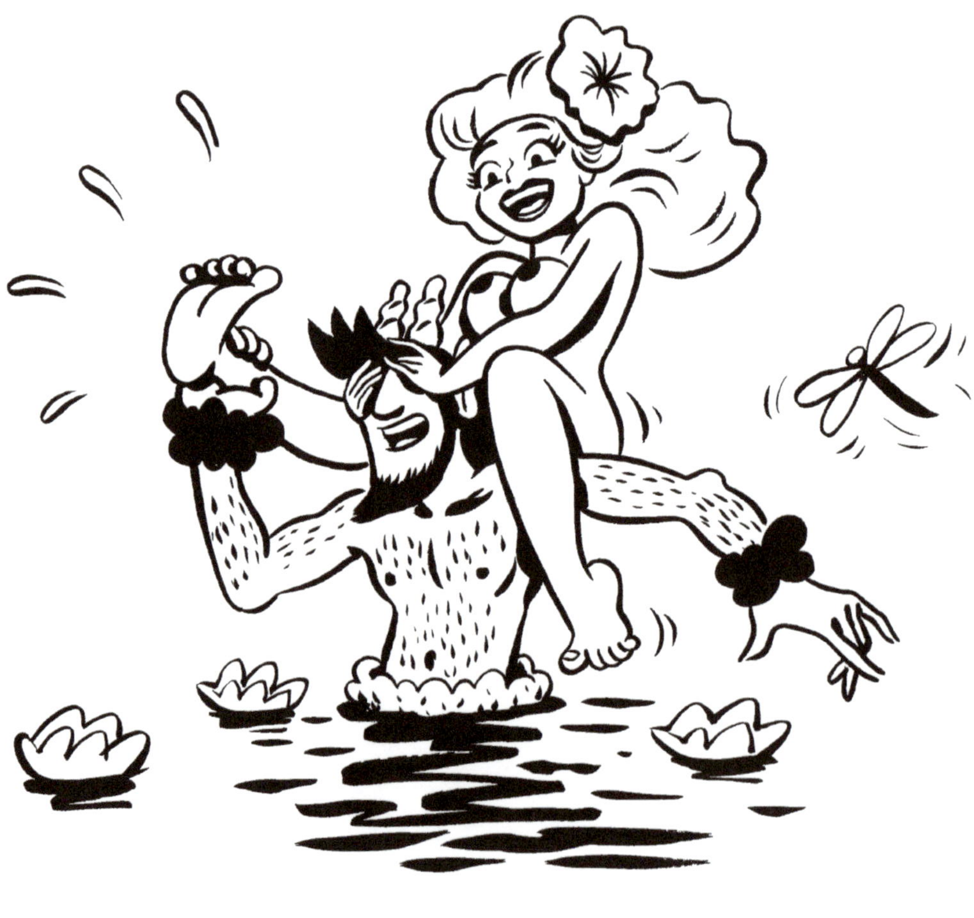

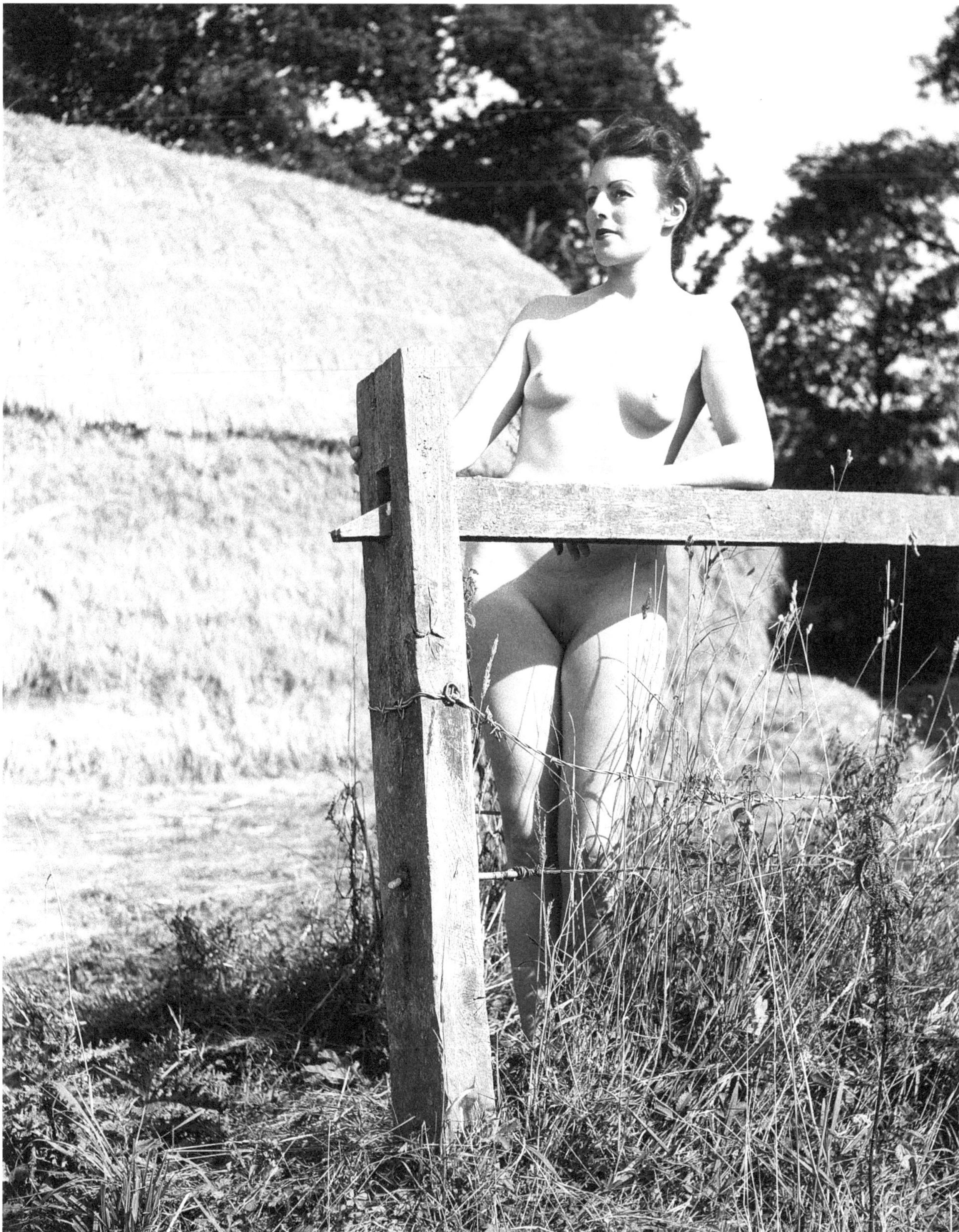

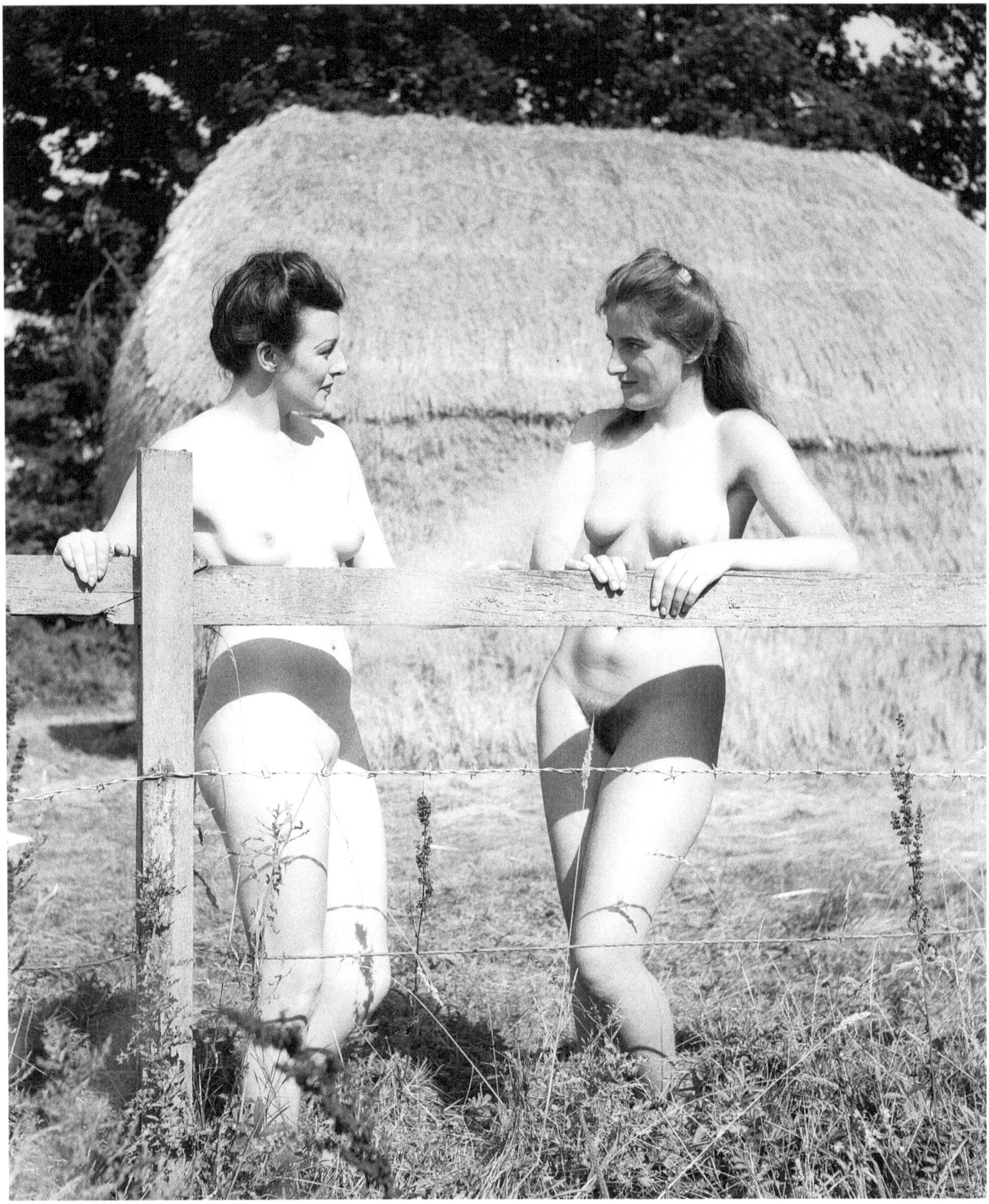

Above: *Sussex Maidens*, "Farmyard Backchat", 1949, page 32. Orginal caption: Naturists are no different from ordinary folk, and these two girls are probably dicussing the latest fashions – trust them!

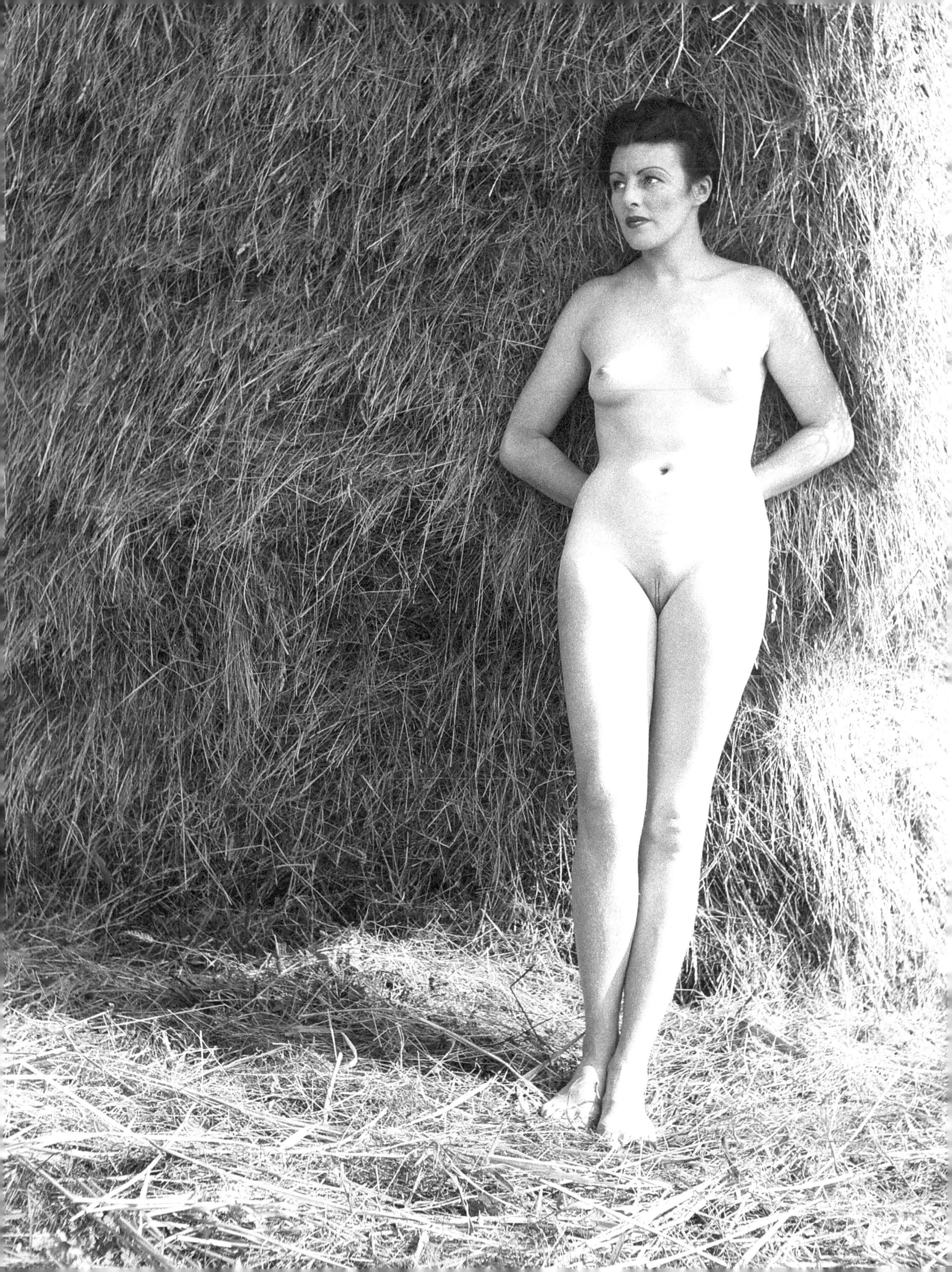

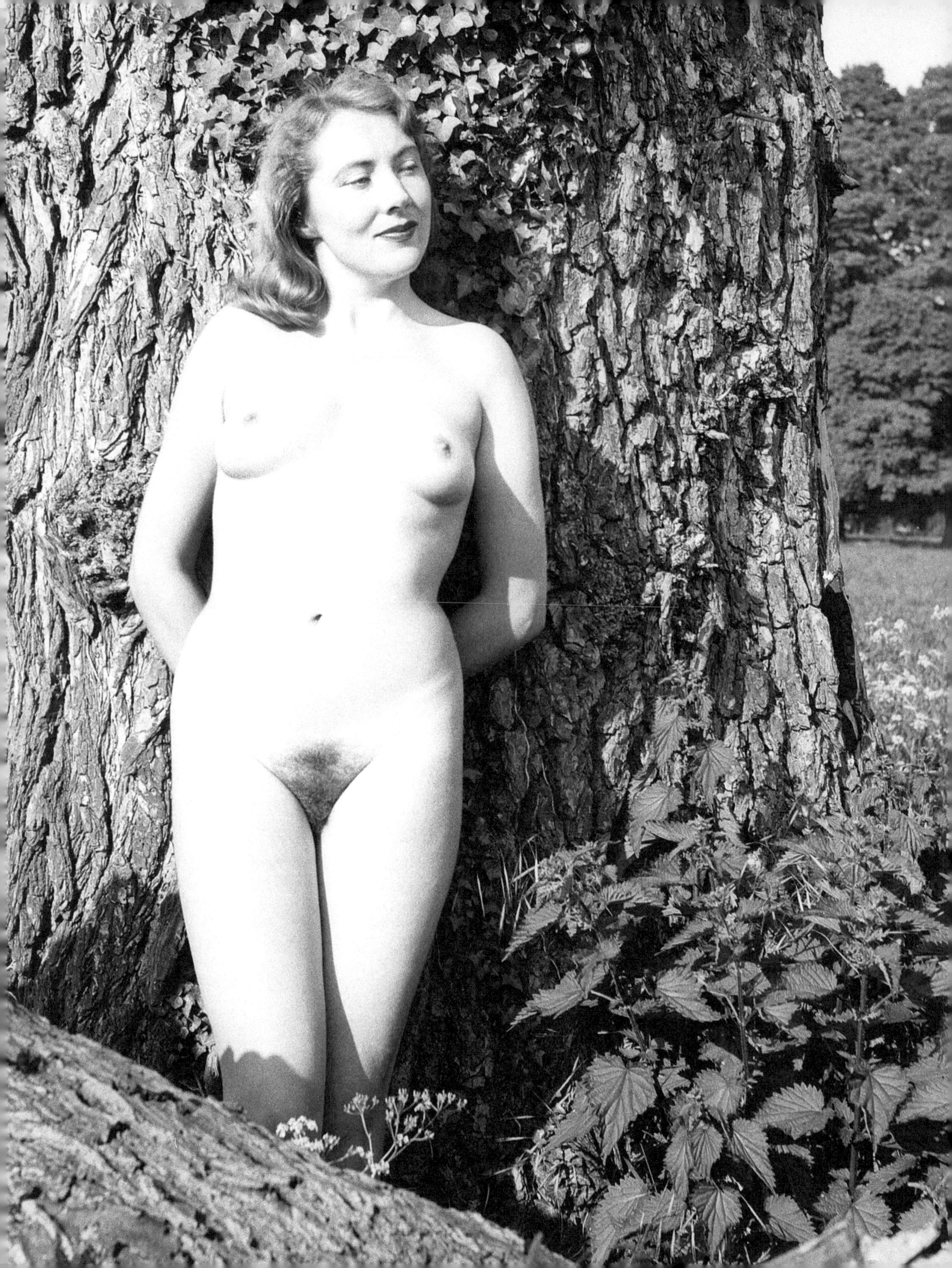

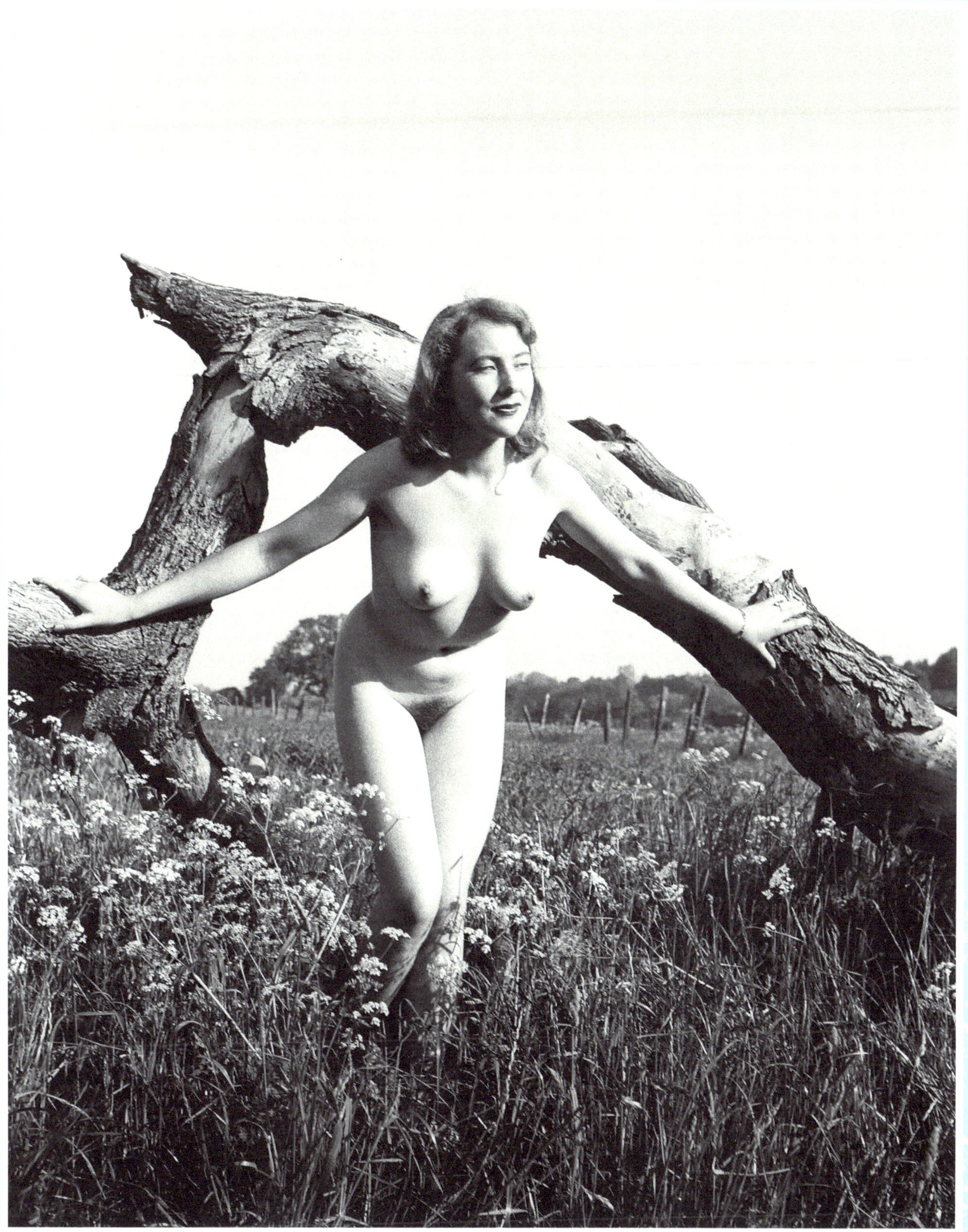

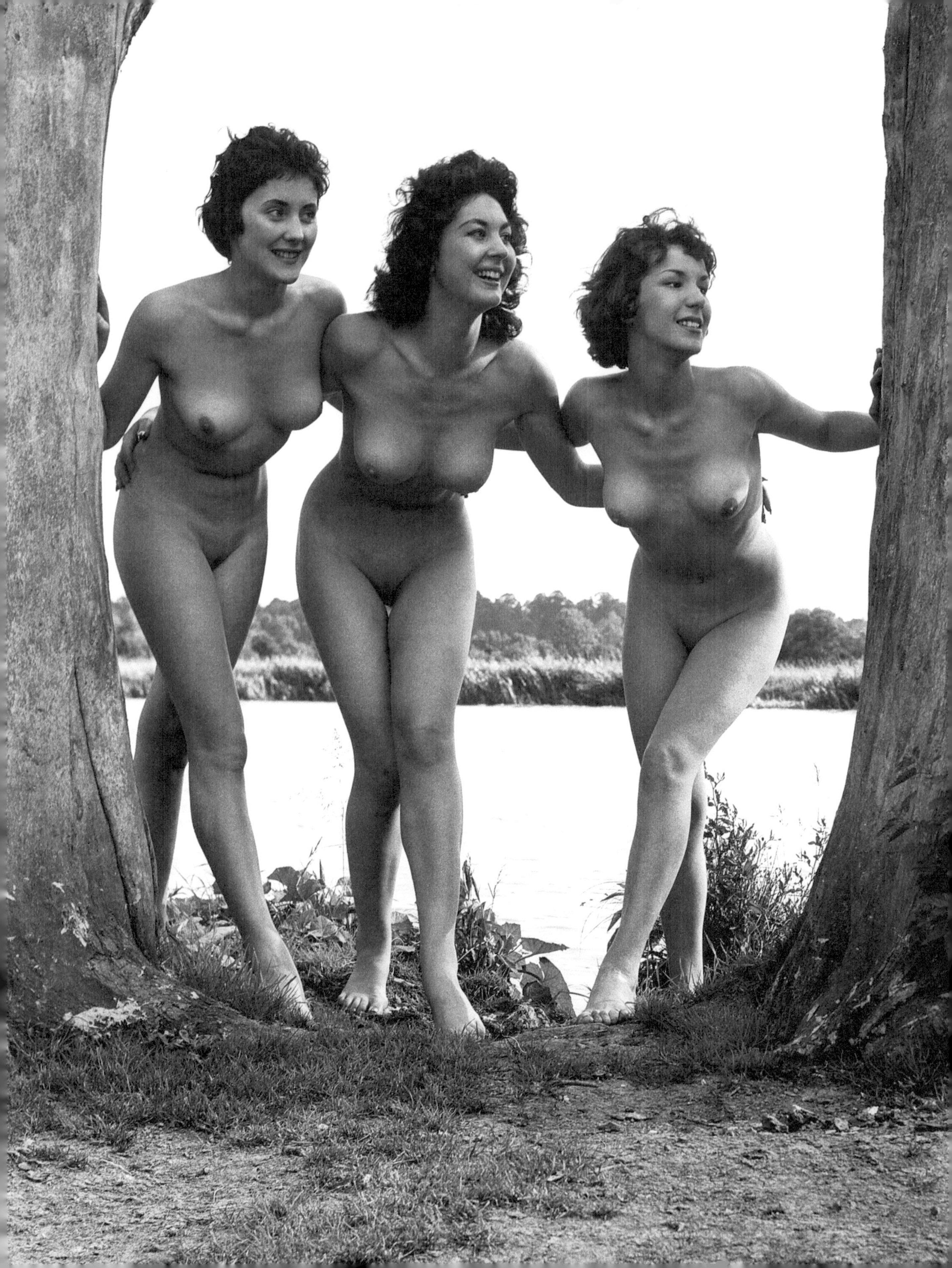

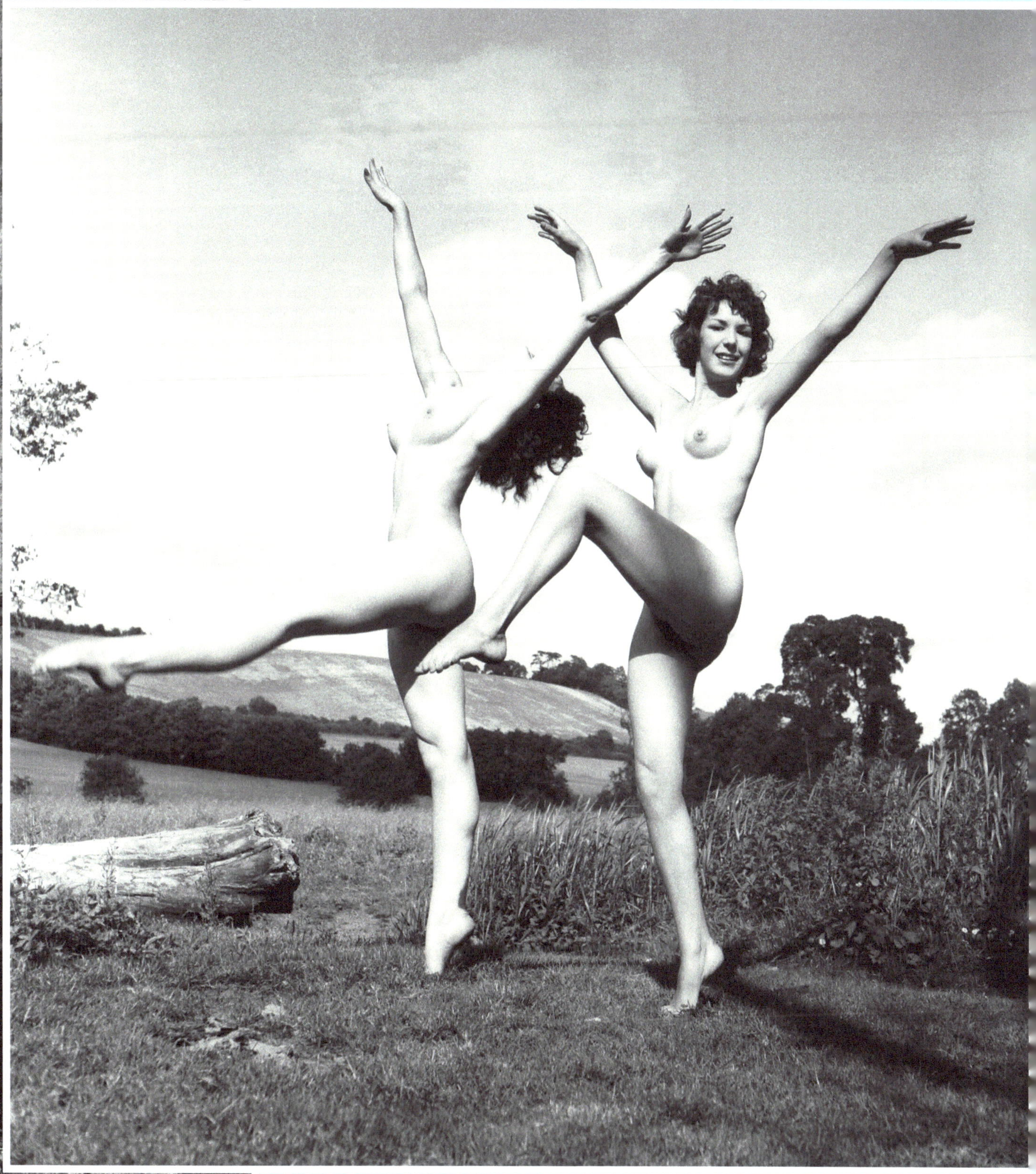

Left: Sherrie Ann Scott, left; Lee Sothern, centre. **Above:** Lee Sothern, left.

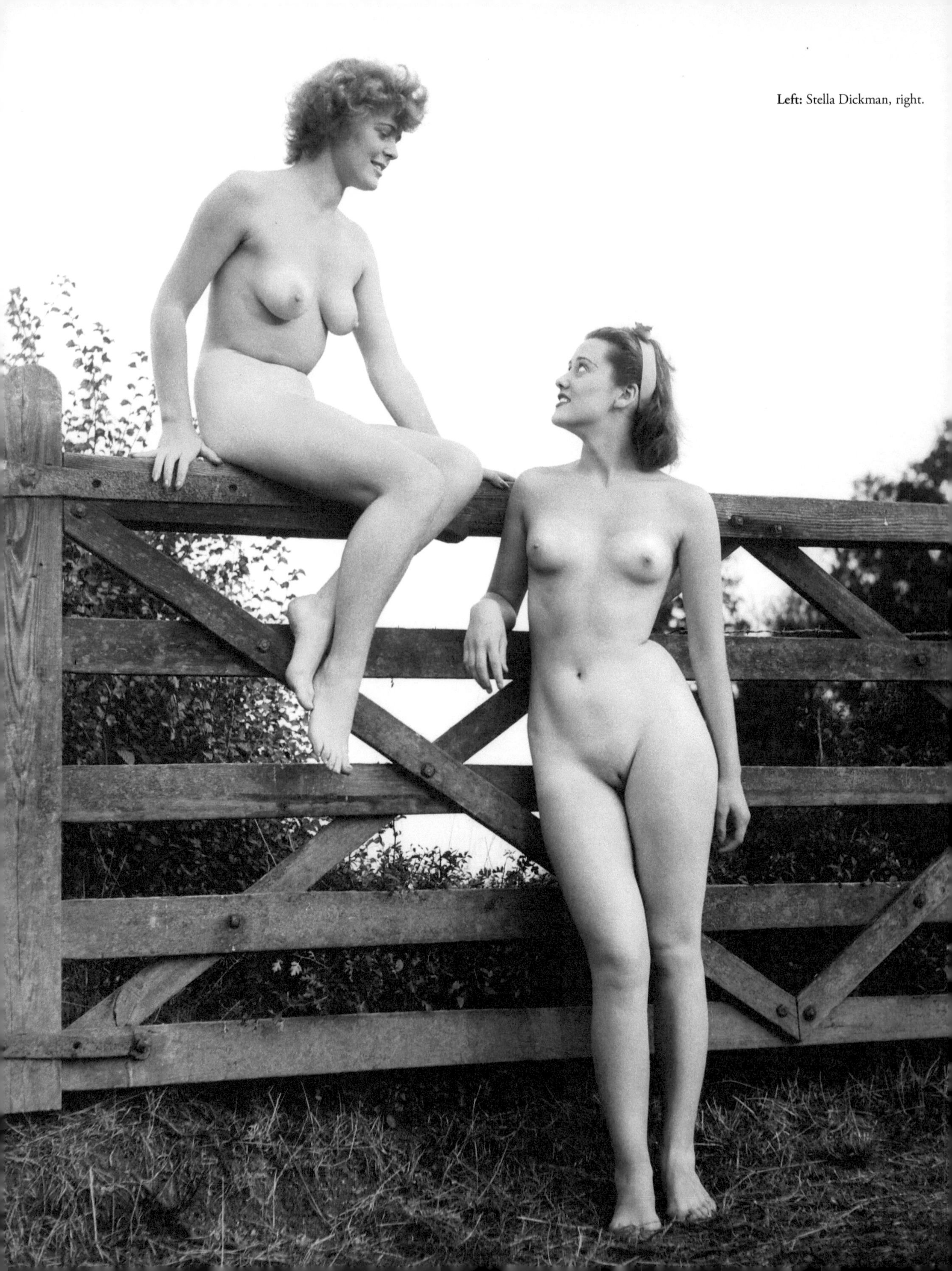

Left: Stella Dickman, right.

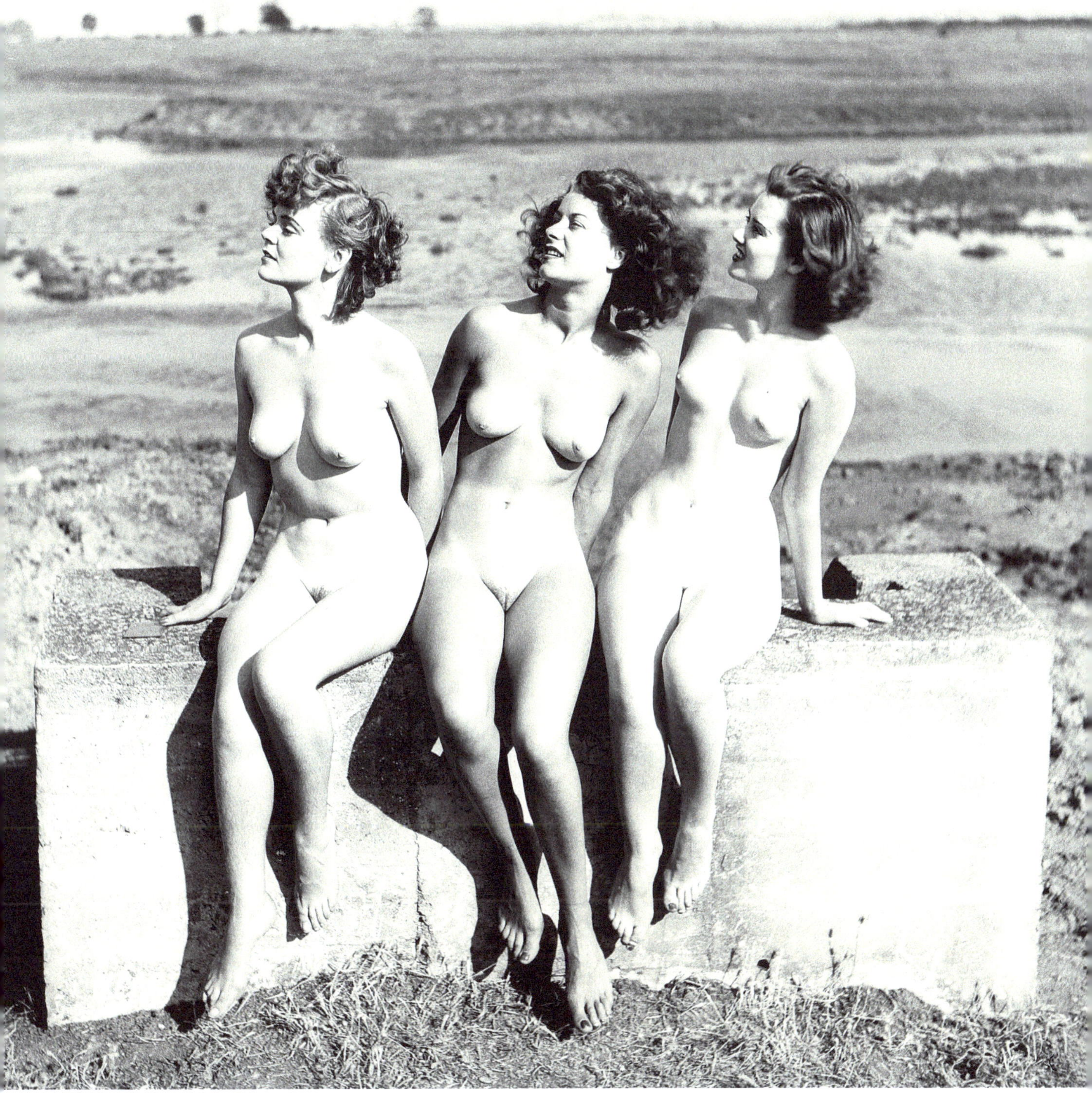

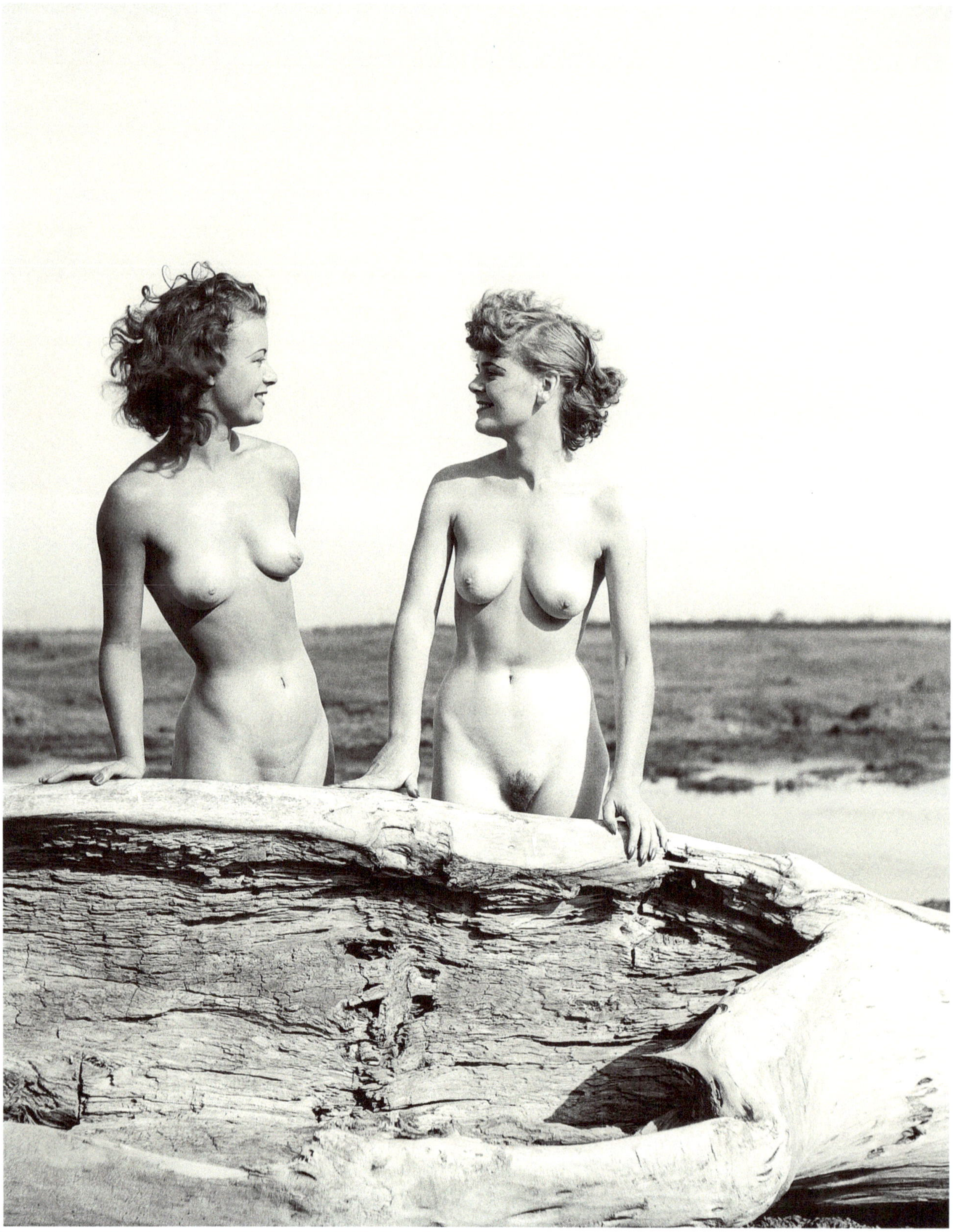

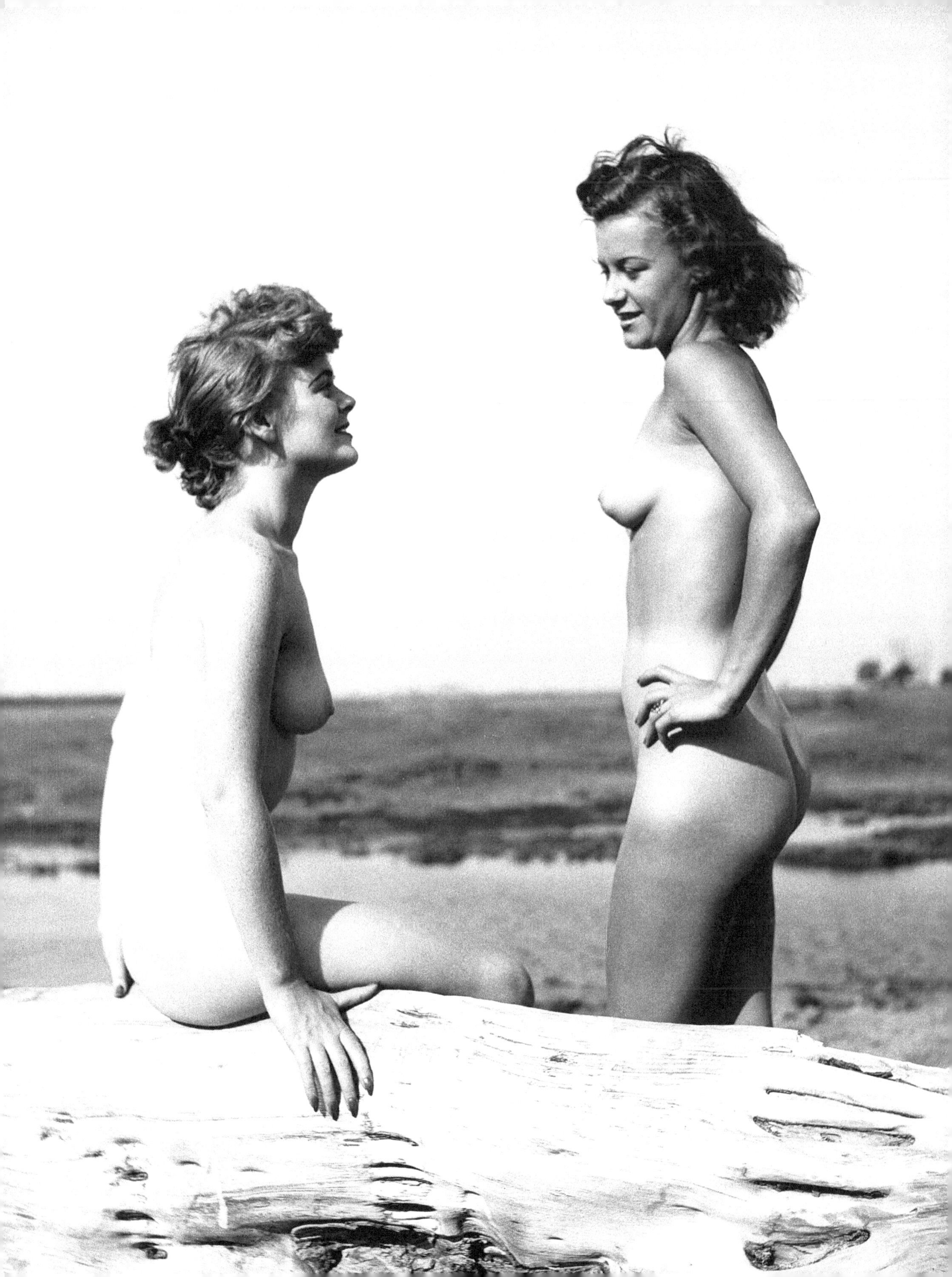

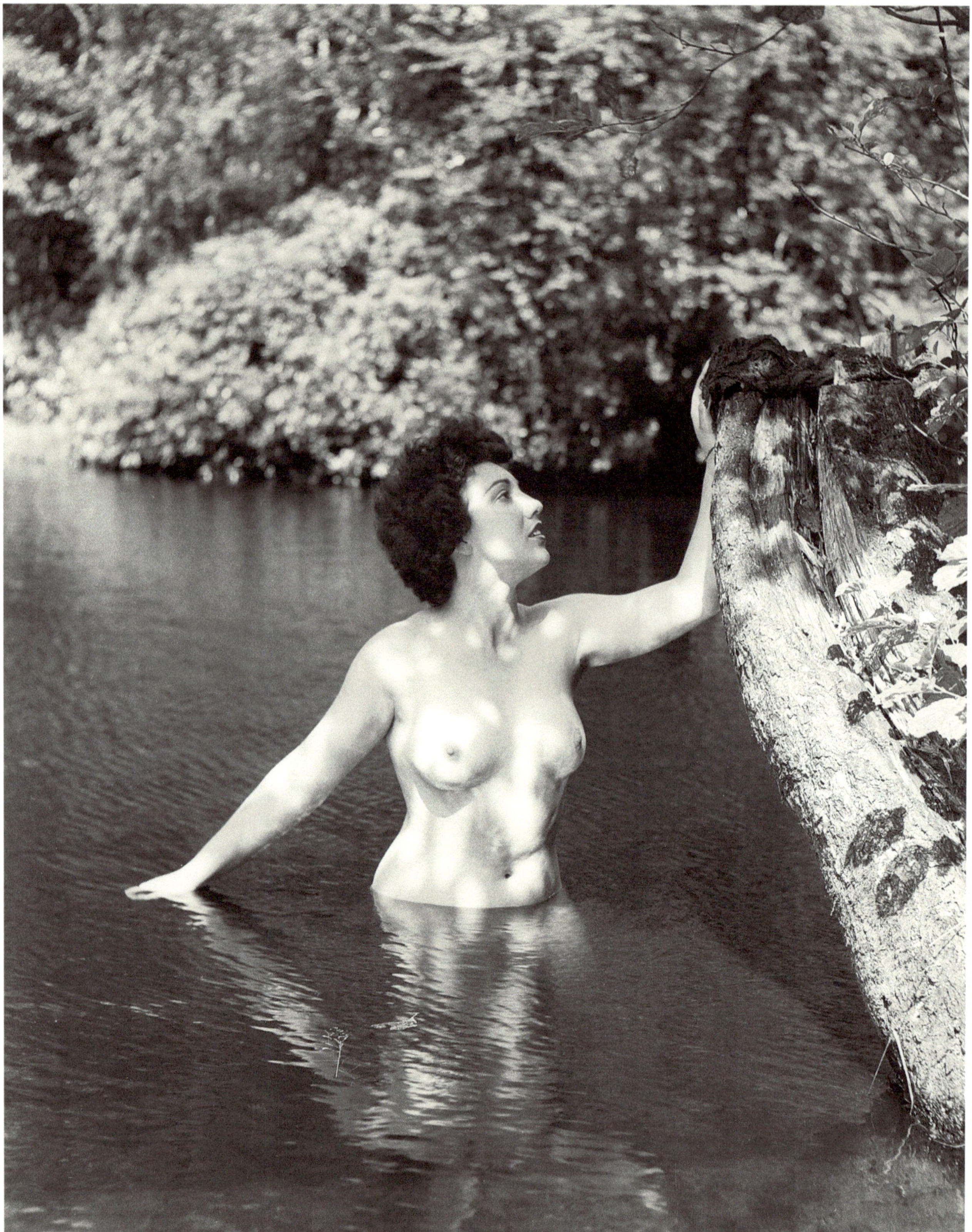

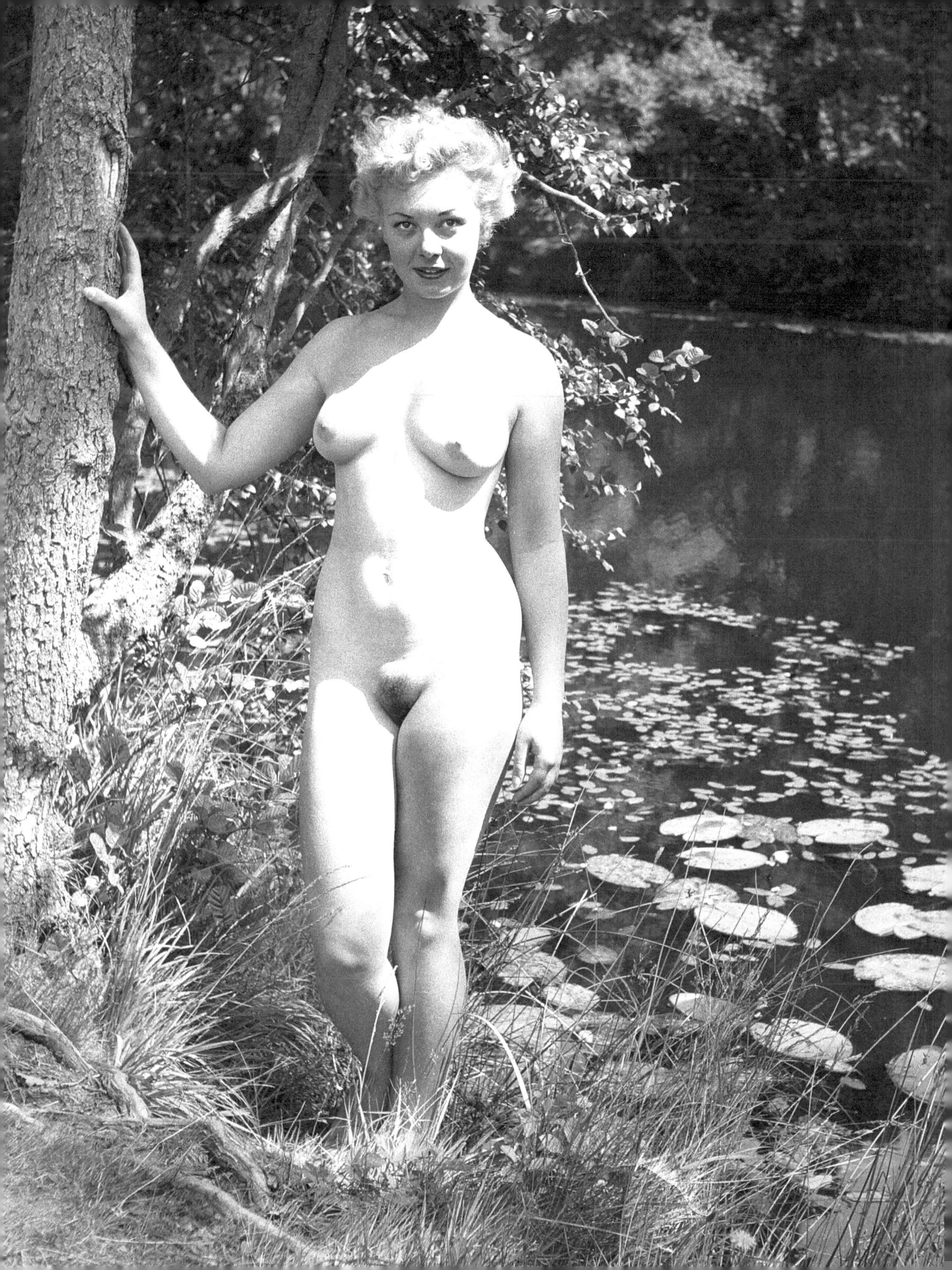

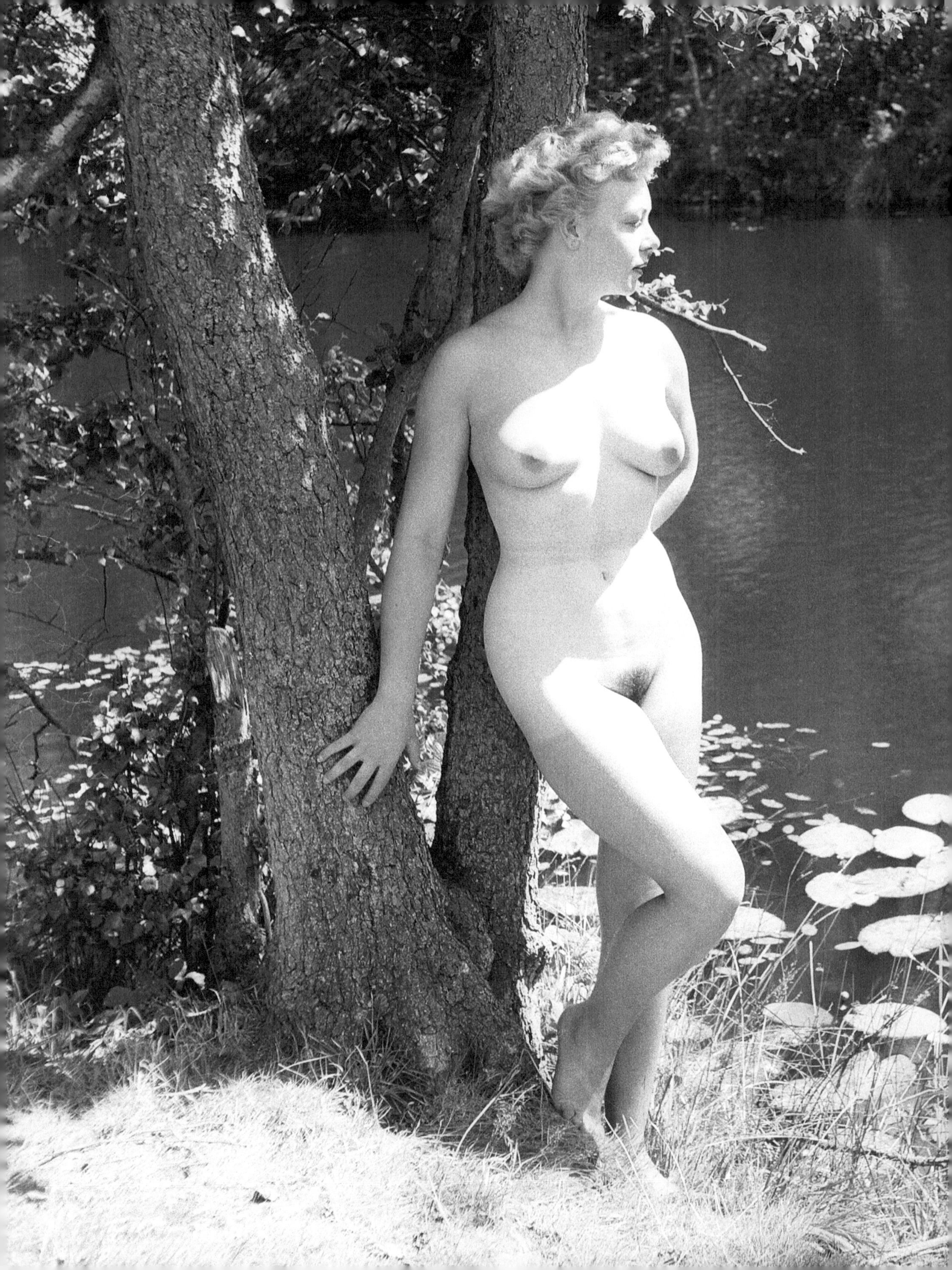

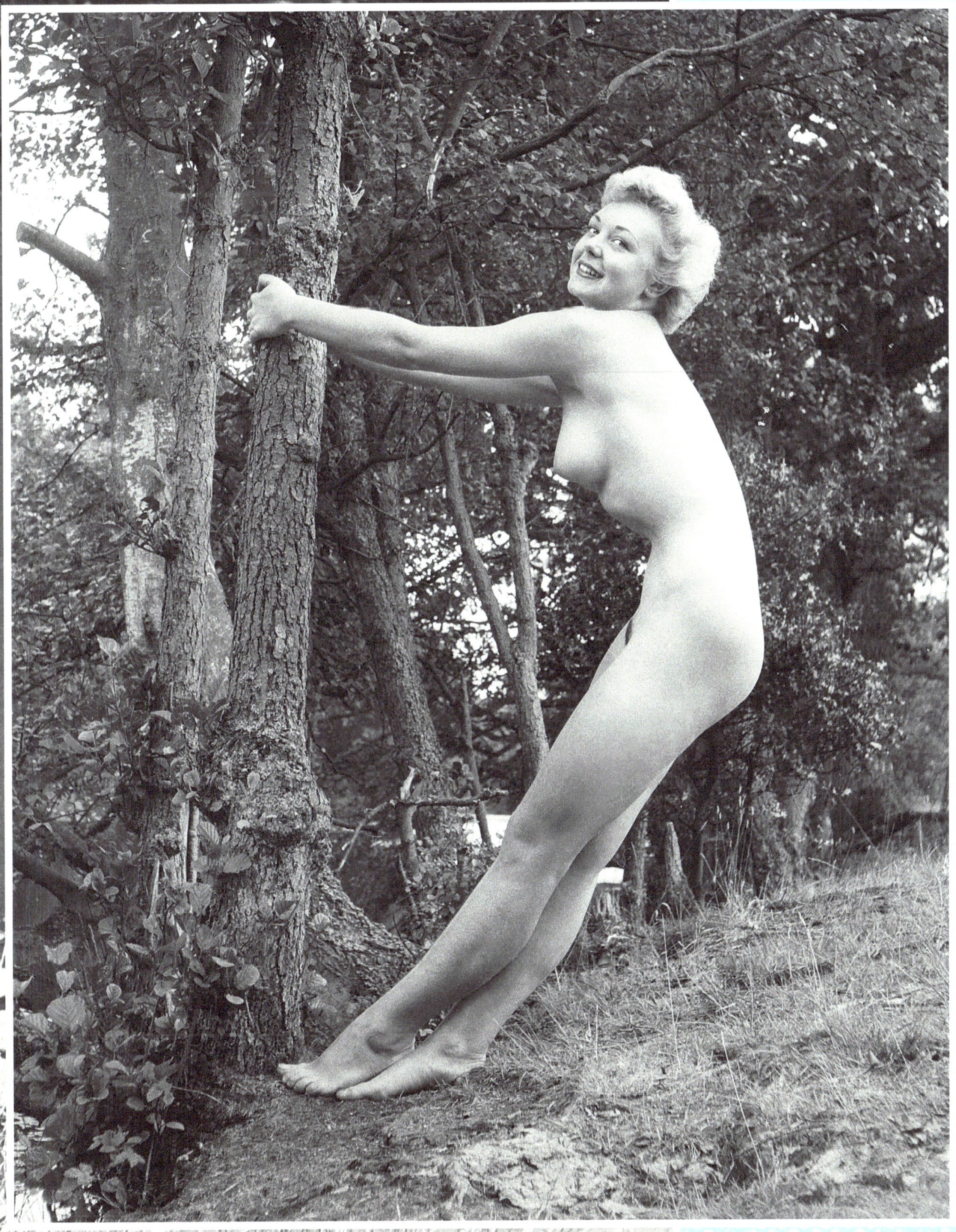

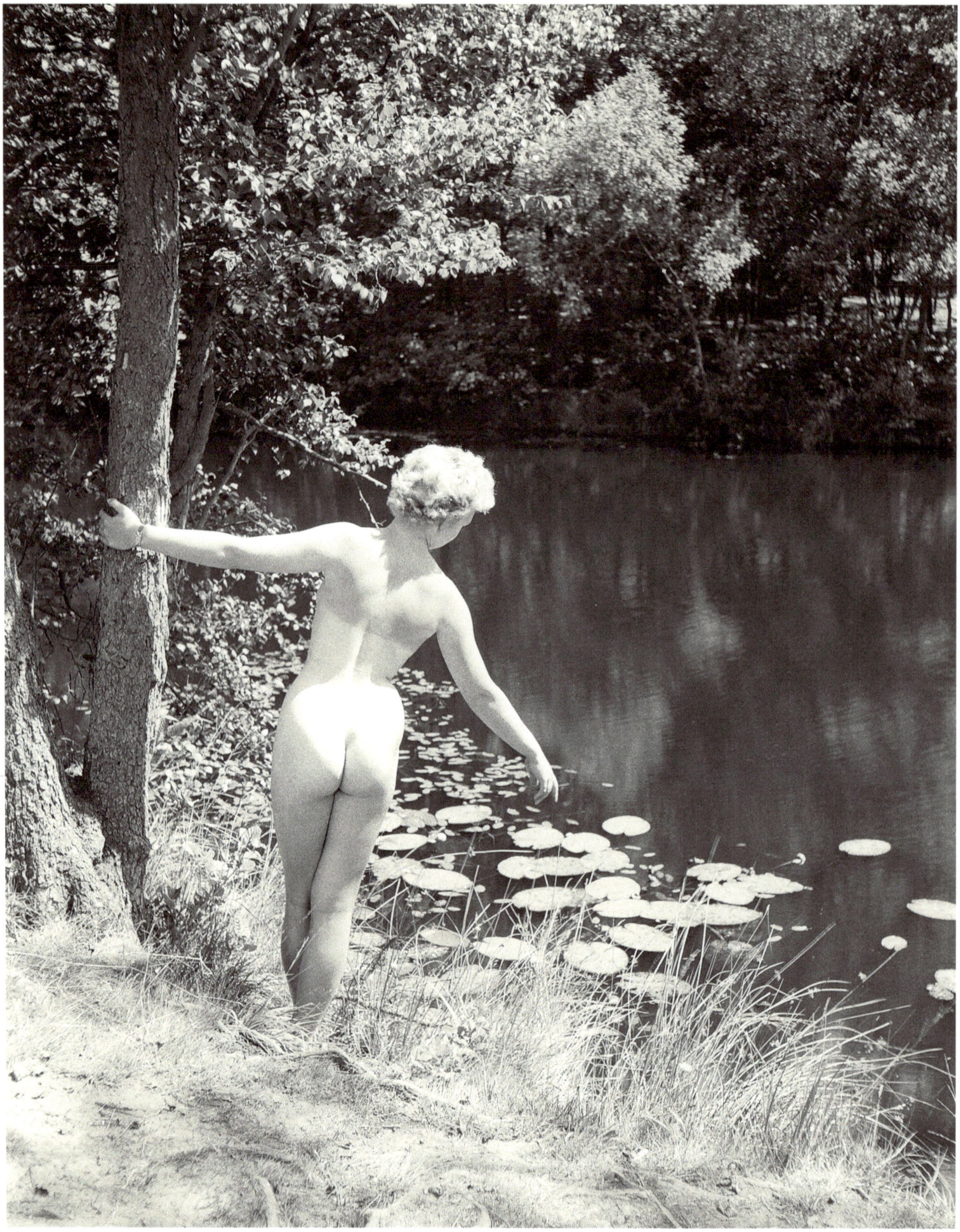

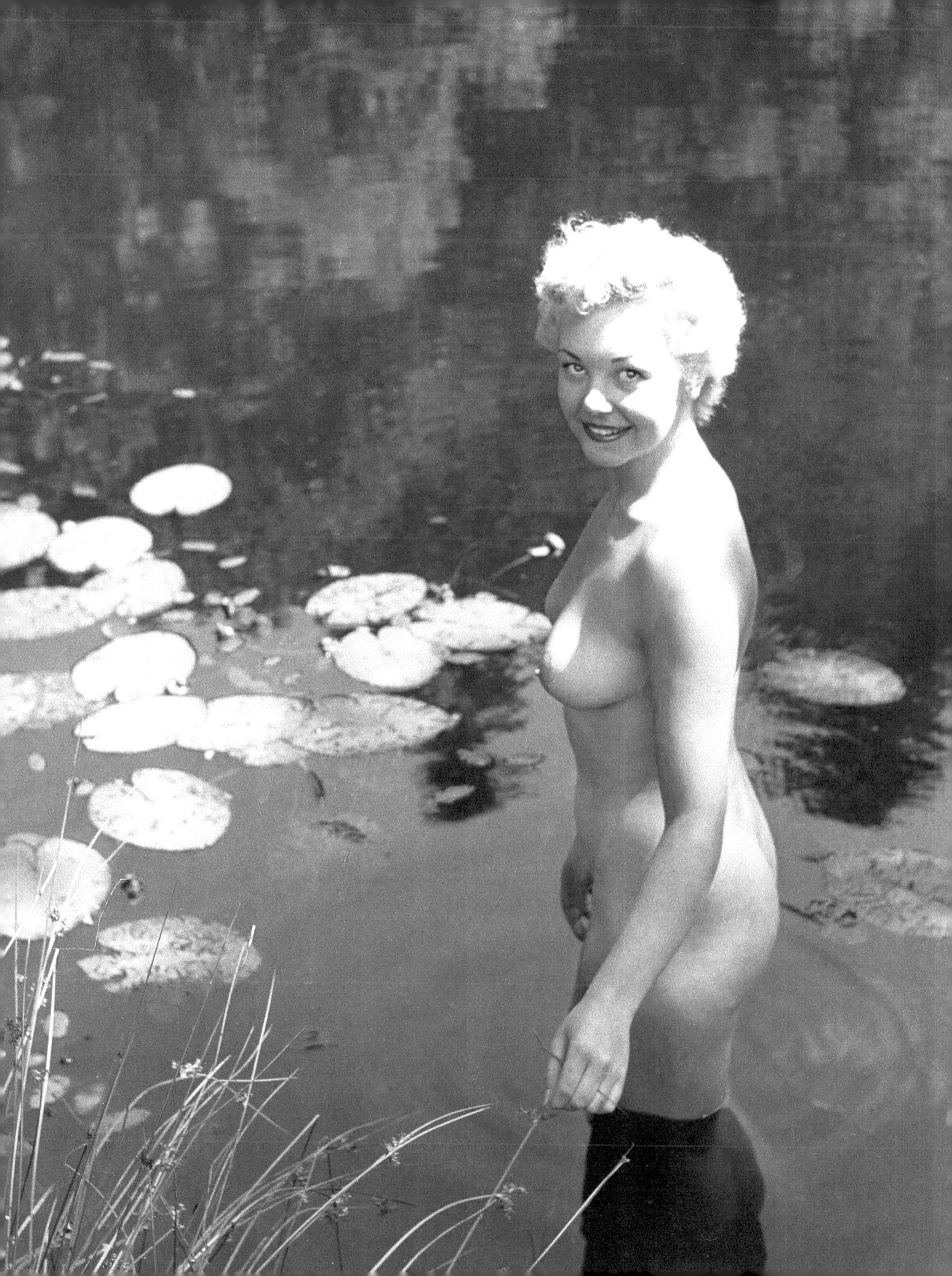

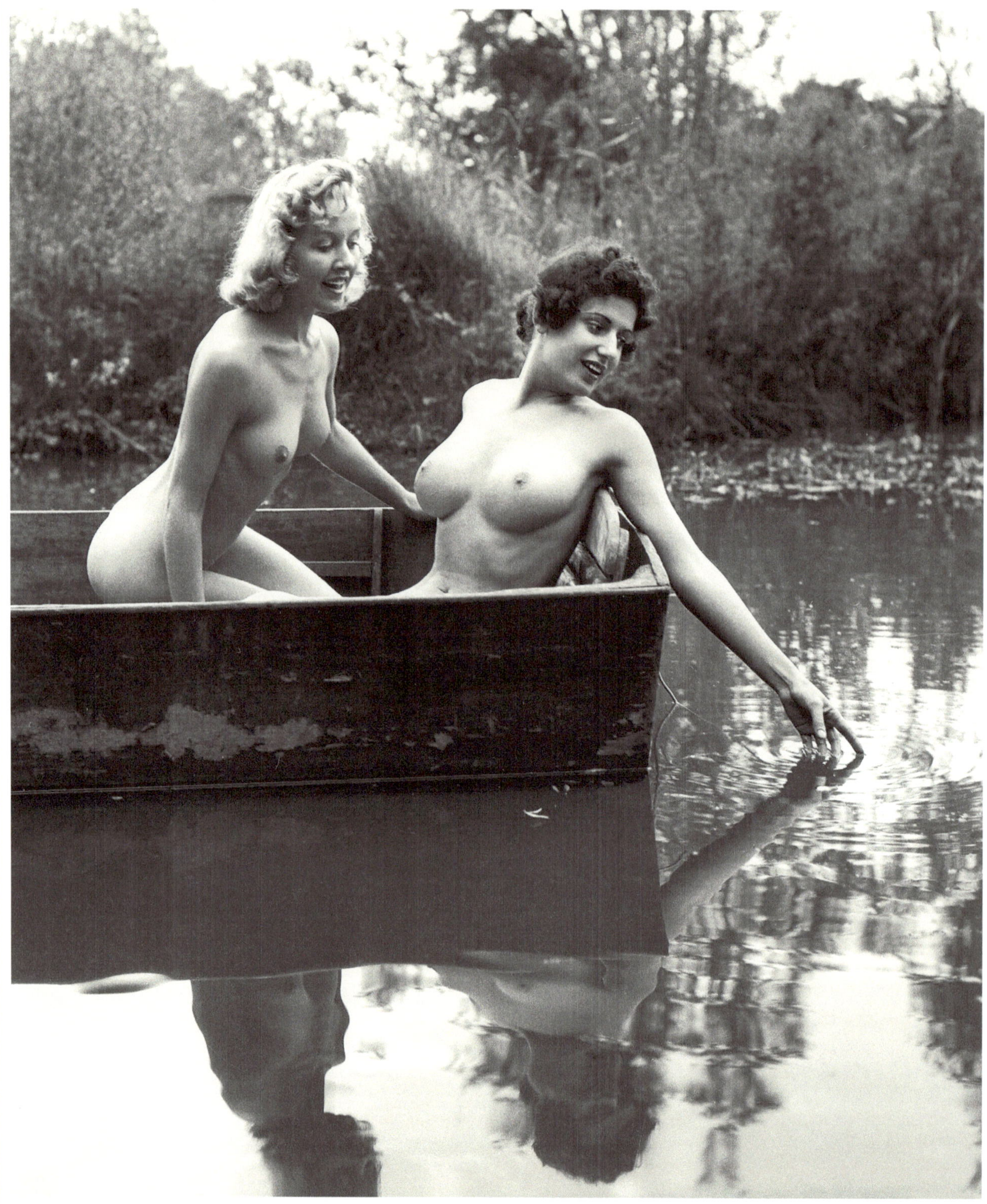

Above: Audrey Wayne, left; Venita Drake, right. **Right:** *Sussex Maidens*, "The Girl Behind the Fence", 1949, page 22. Model: Adrienne Germaine. Original caption: An attractive glimpse of "the girl next door" and an unusually revealing "screen".

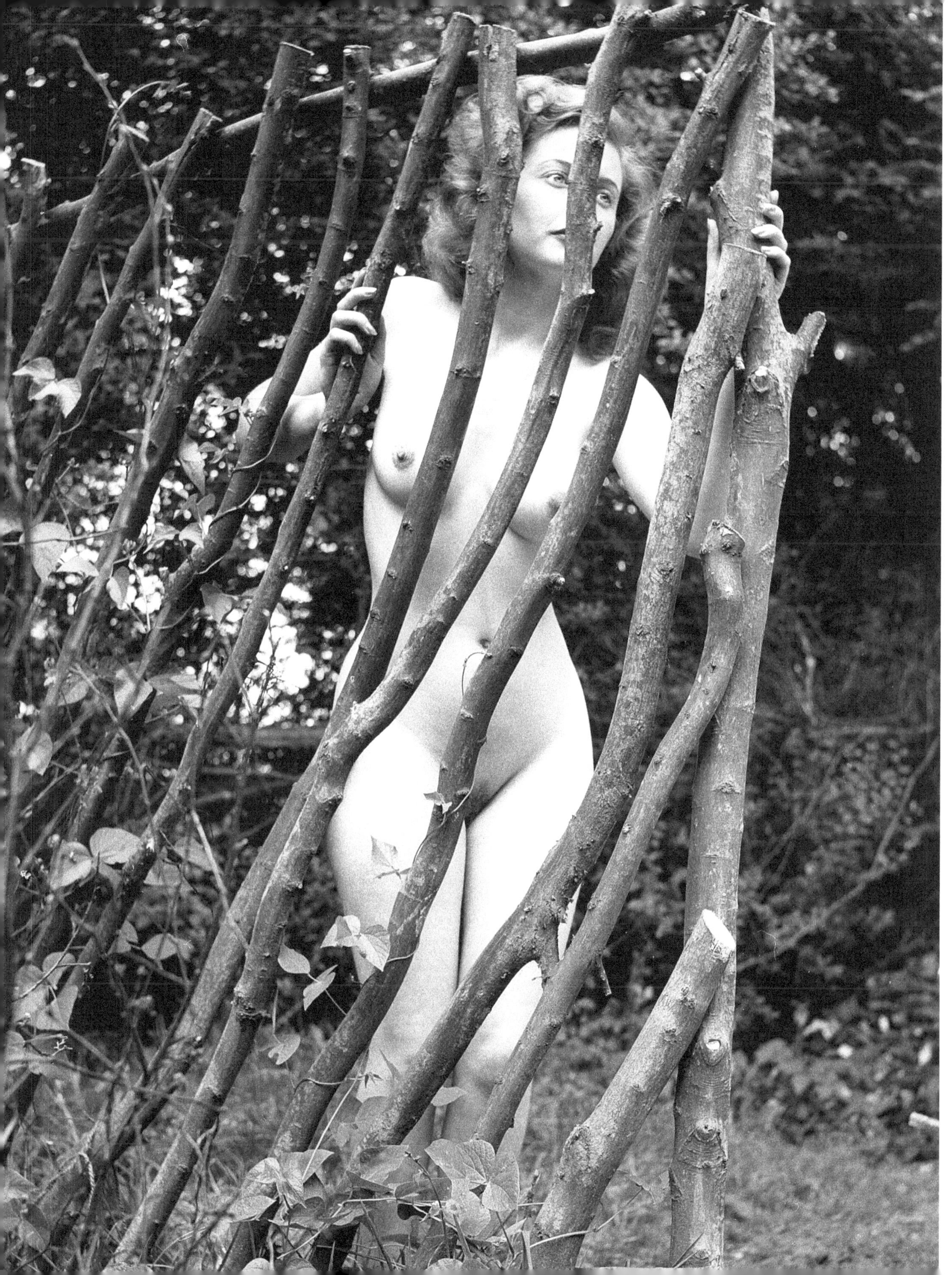

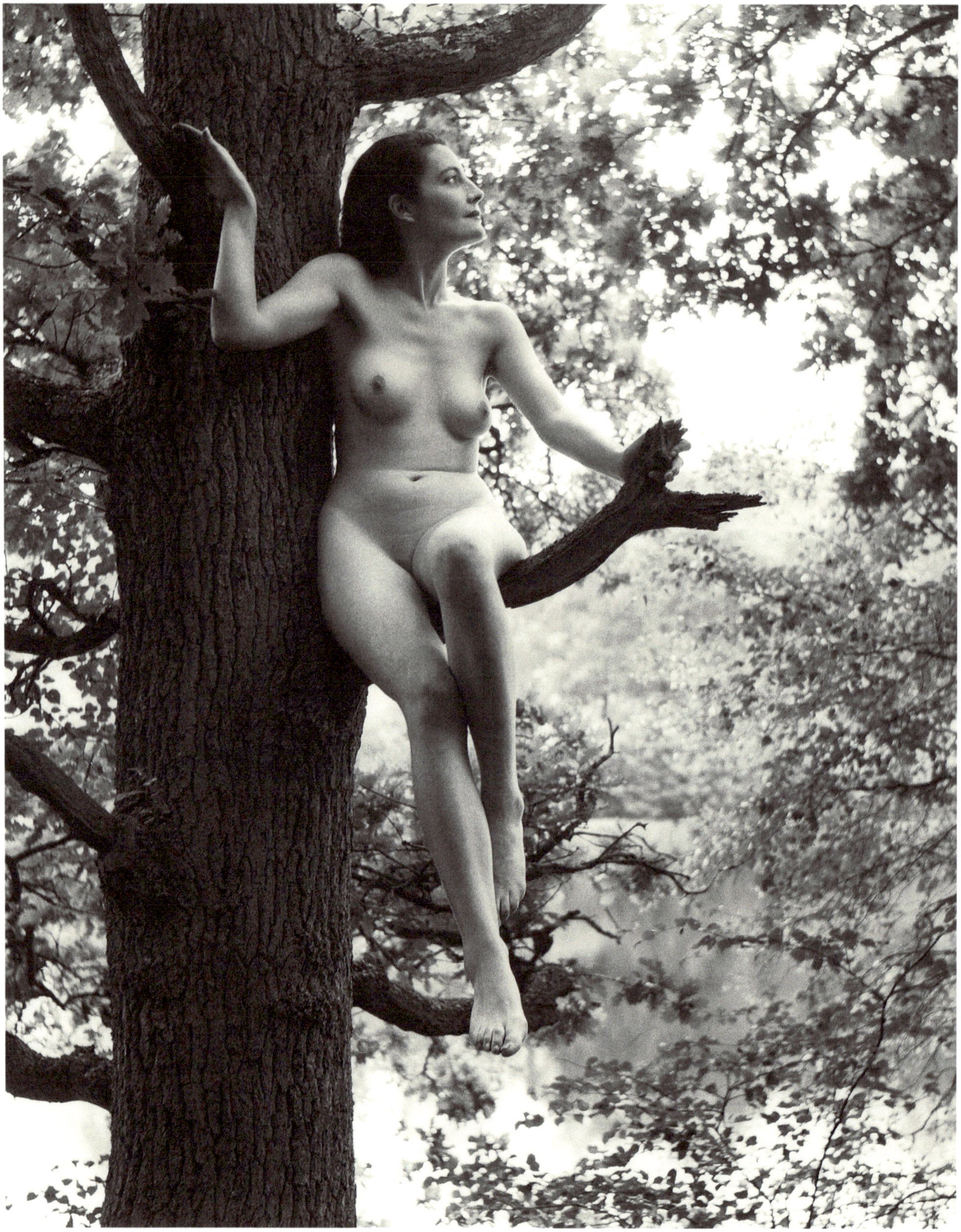

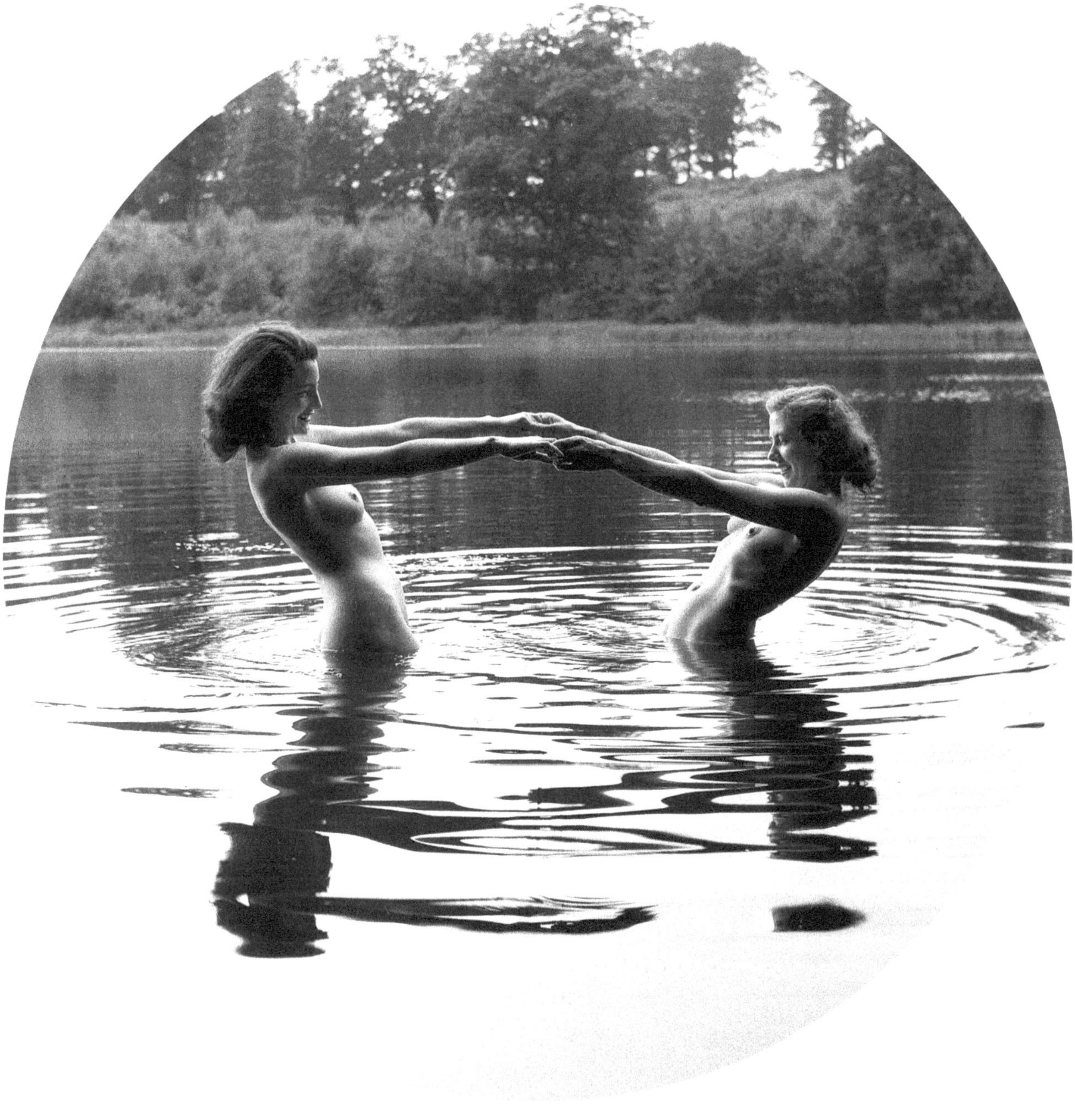

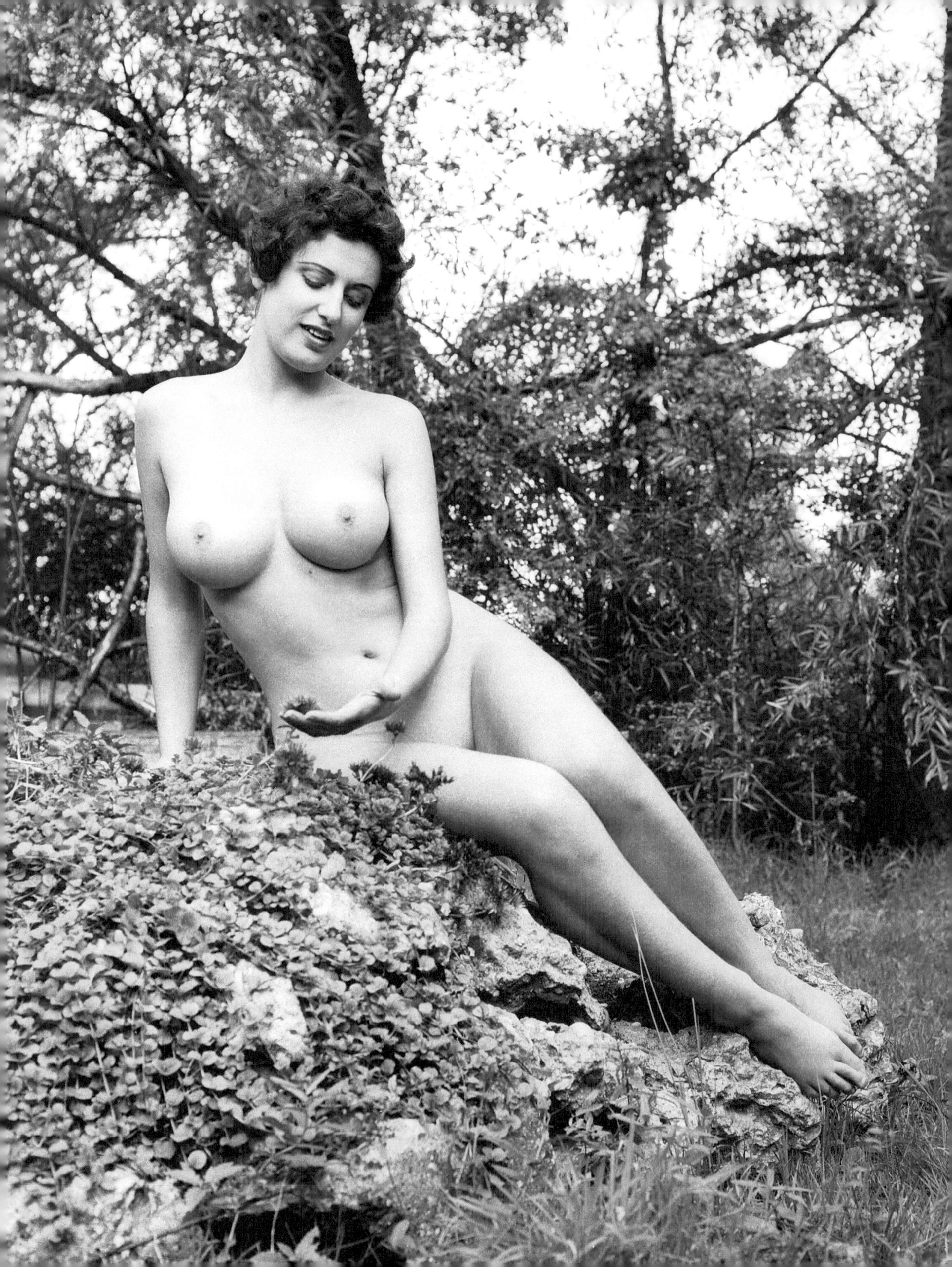

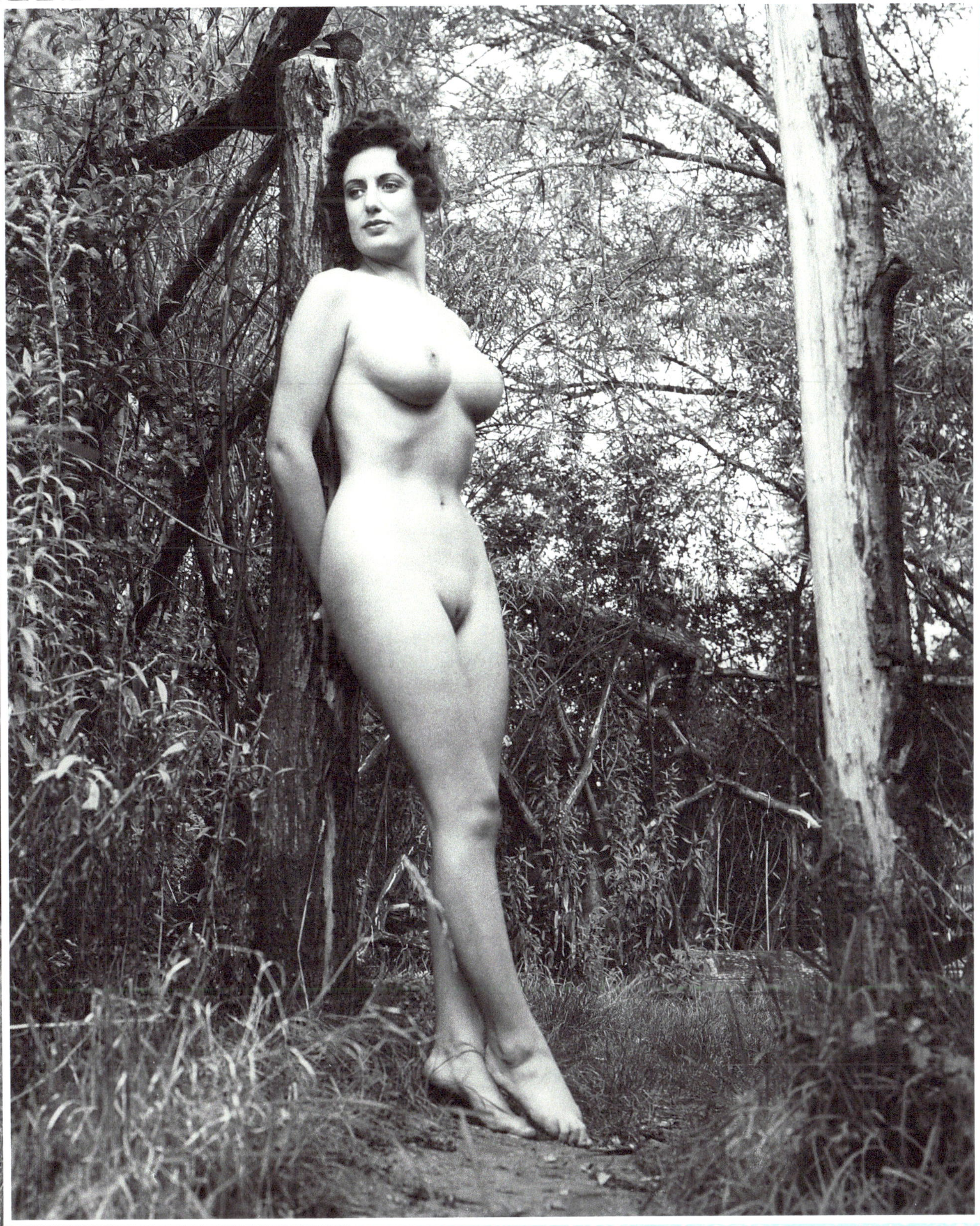

Left and above: Full-time model and glamour girl Venita Drake.

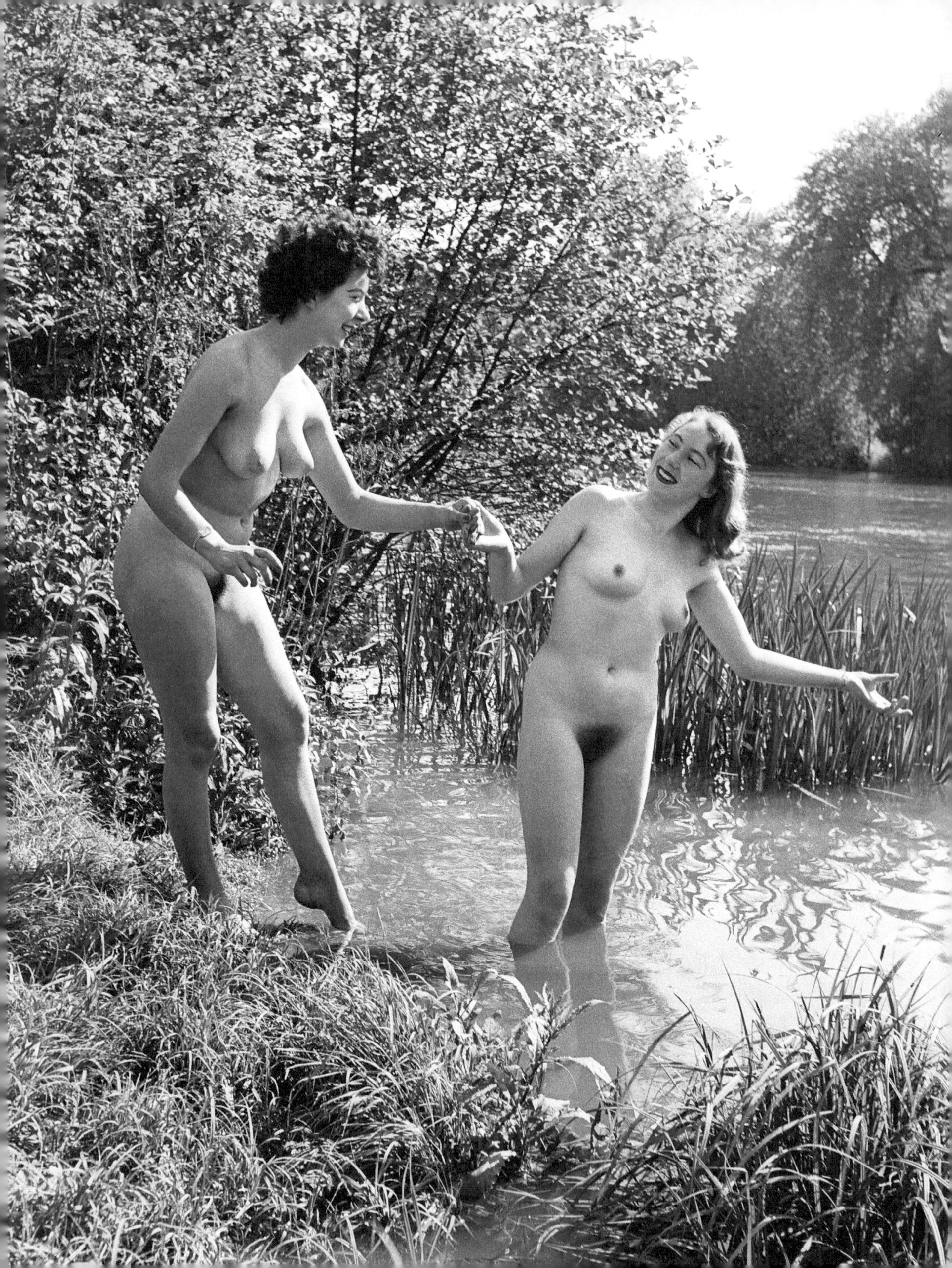

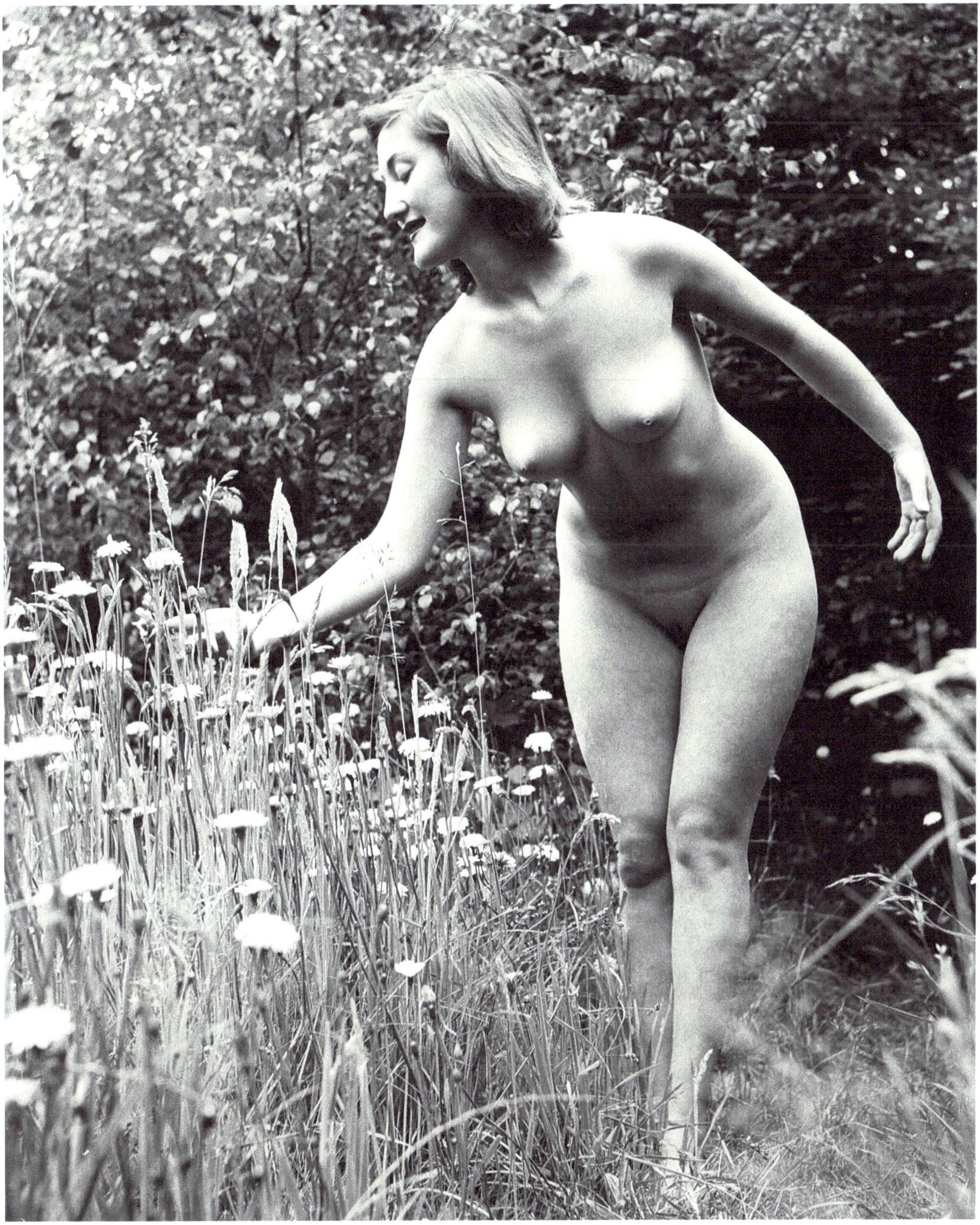

Above: Barbara Thourgood.

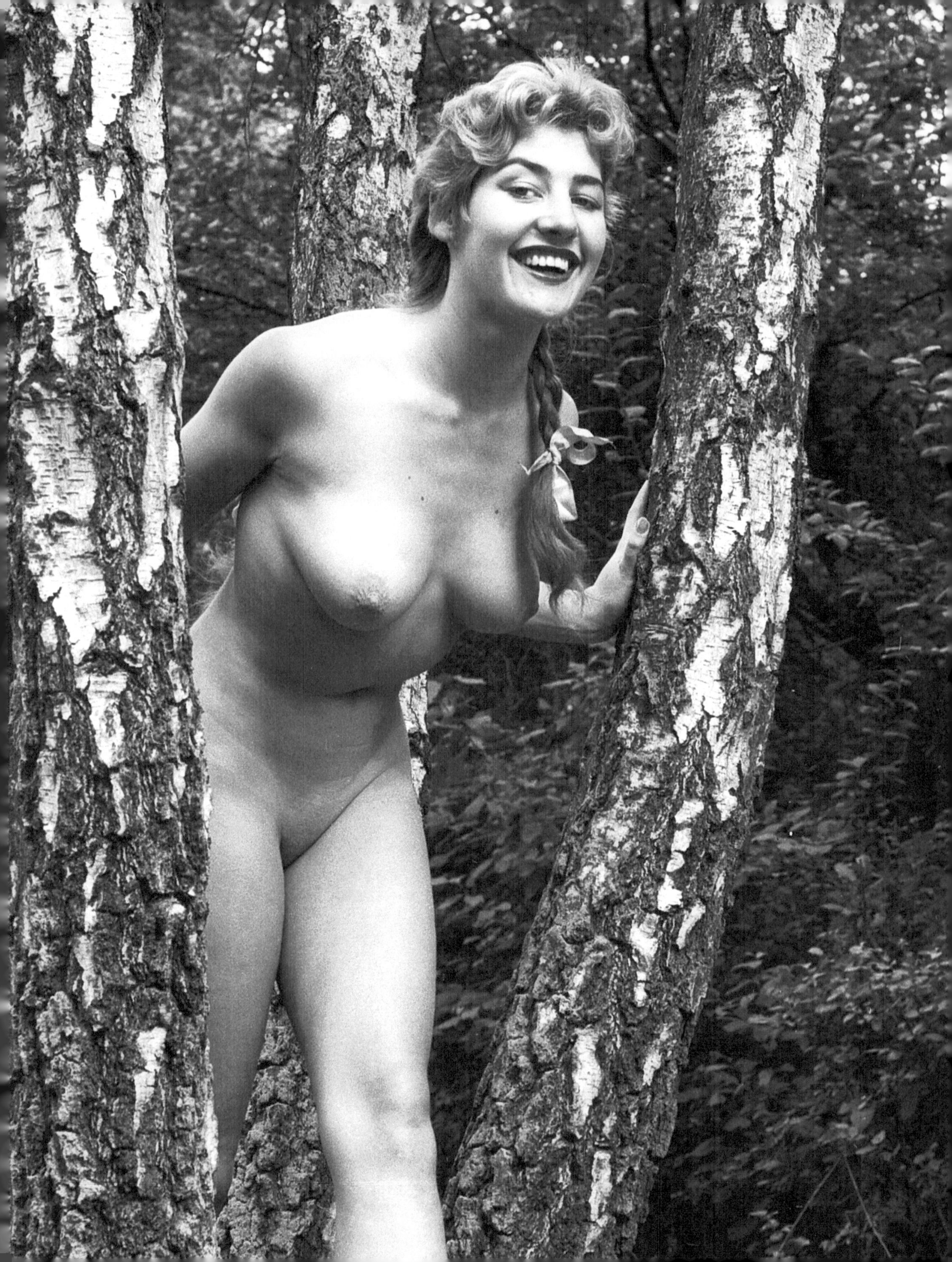

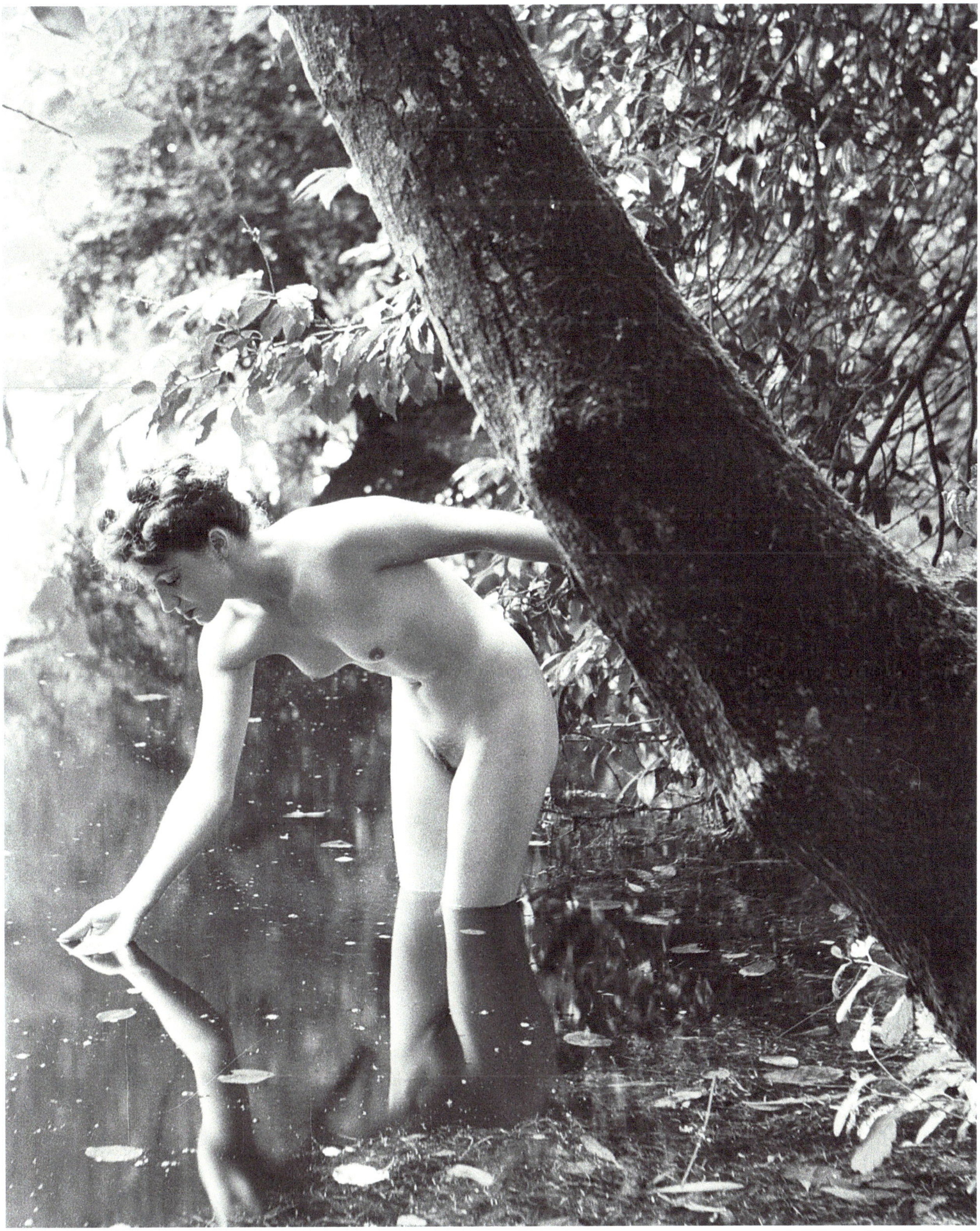

Left: Nancy Roberts.

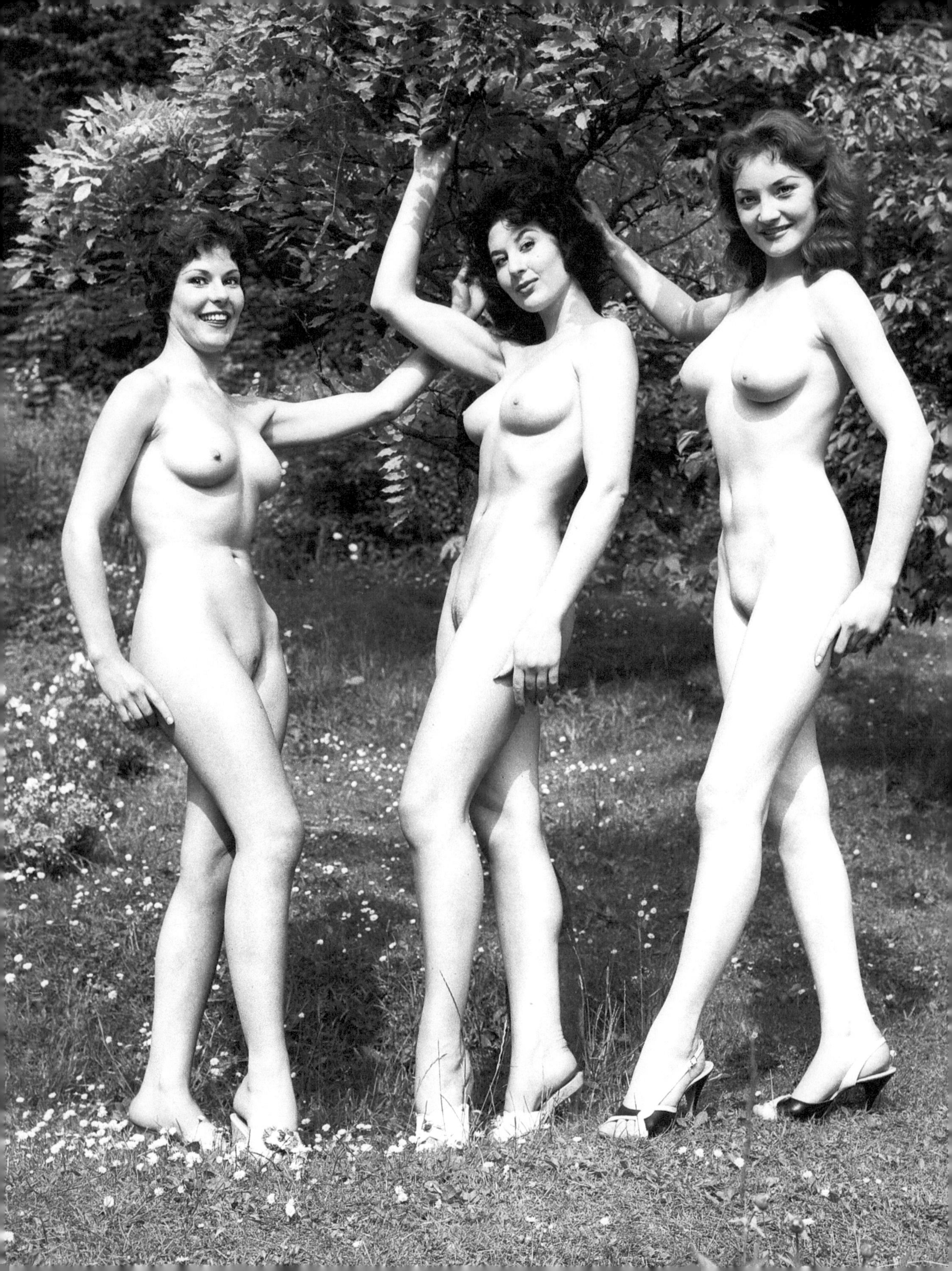

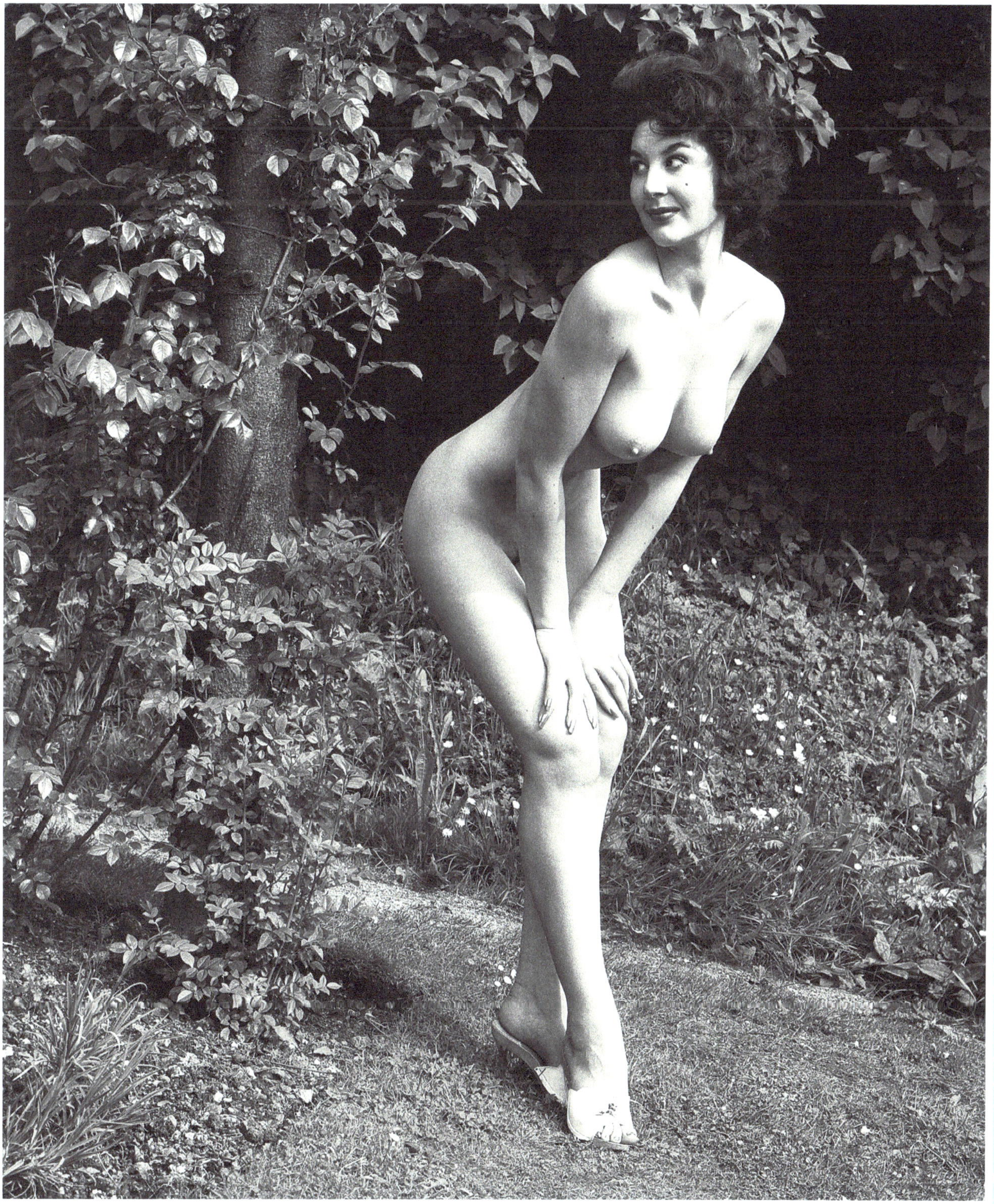

Left: June Russell, Lee Sothern (aka Grace Jackson), and Carole Richards. June Russell, like Lee Sothern, regularly posed for the notorious George Harrison Marks. She lived in Sutton in Surrey and in 1960 starred in the Aqua-revue at Bournemouth. **Above:** Lee Sothern.

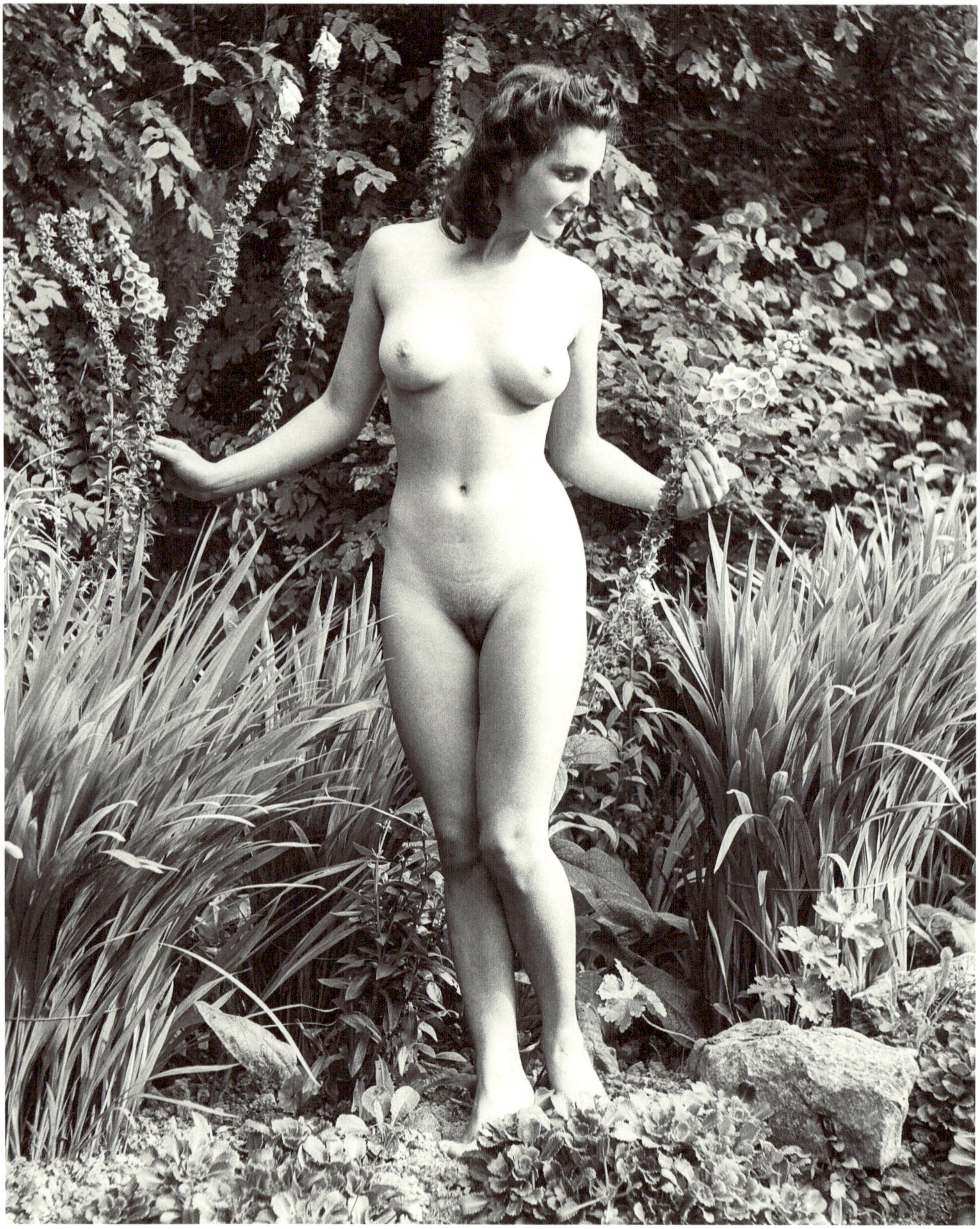

Above: Audrey Goodman. **Right:** Jill Higgs.

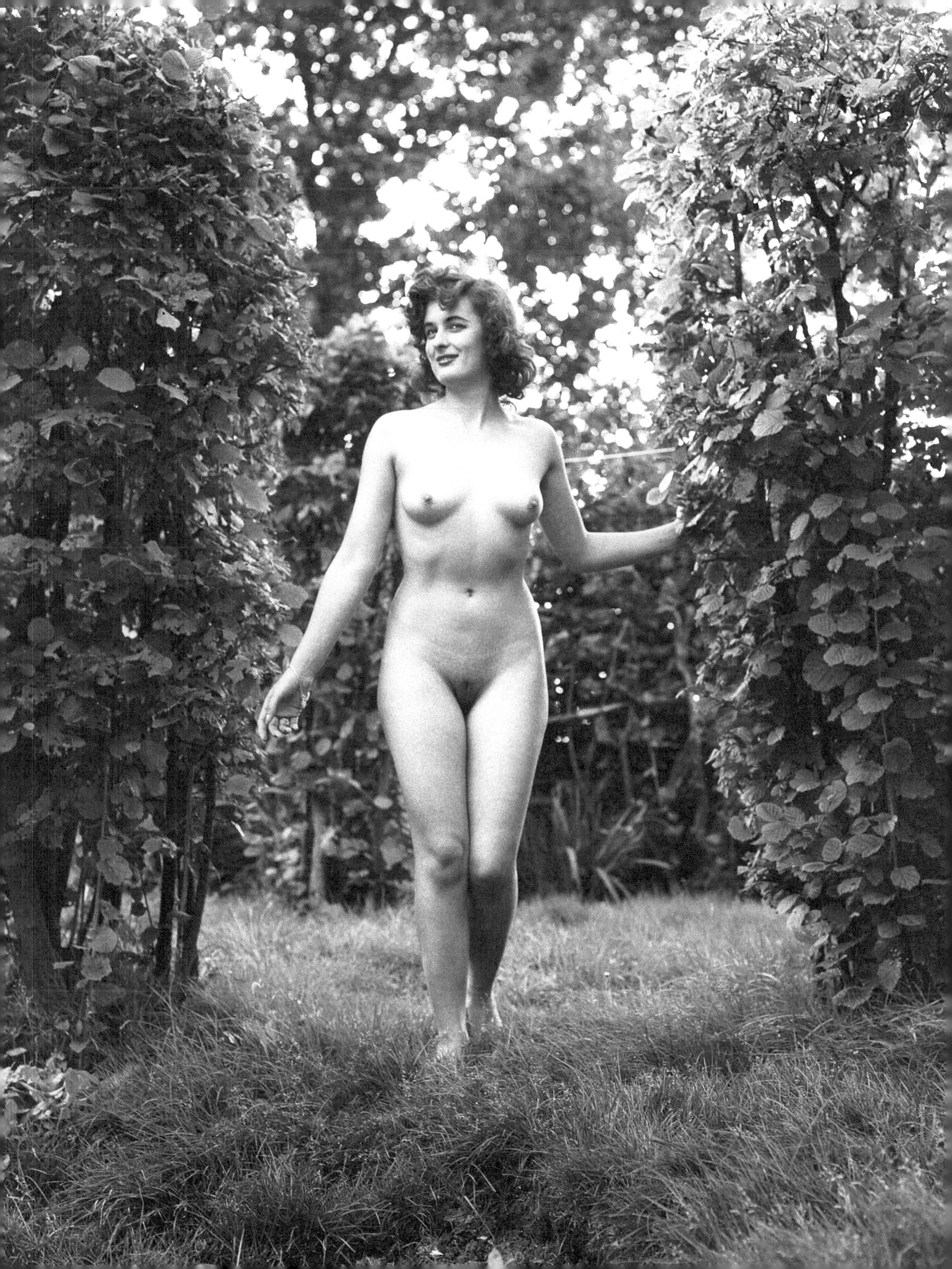

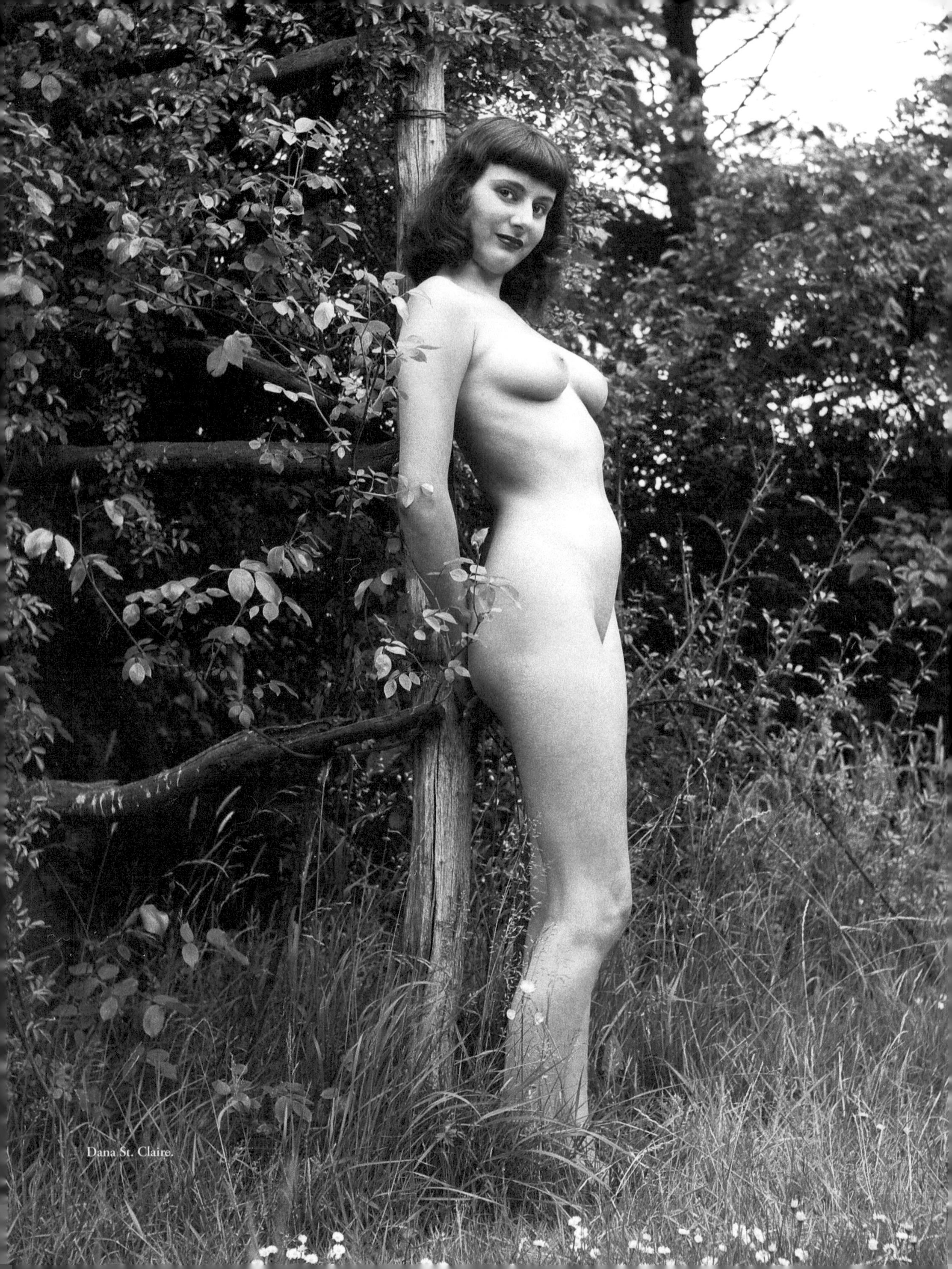

Dana St. Claire.

AVAILABLE TITLES FROM WOLFBAIT

Doing Rude Things
The history of the British sex film.

NEW! **Cinema au Naturel**
A history of nudist film.

Miniten: Rules of the Game
Invented in the 1930s, Miniten is a tennis-like game played by naturists.

Naked as Nature Intended
The epic tale of a nudist picture by Pamela Green, with photographs by Douglas "Dambuster" Webb, DFM.

The Naked Truth About Harrison Marks
The notorious biography by Franklyn Wood.

Past Masters of the Nude
An illustrated bibliography of nude photography books published in England from 1896 to 1960.

THE STEPHEN GLASS COLLECTION

Amazons of Yesteryear
A rare, action-packed collection of images of wrestling women of the 1940s and 1950s.

Beauty Off-Duty
Relaxed, everyday moments caught on camera.

Naked in the Menagerie
A playful look at Eve accompanied by her animal friends.

Nudist Camp Follies – volumes 1 and 2
An intimate look at the natural and free atmosphere in Sun Clubs.

Nymphs and Naiads
Beauty unadorned and outdoors.

NEW! **Poise and Pose**
A magnificent series of photographs of female beauty taken in the studio.

Order online at wolfbait.co.uk

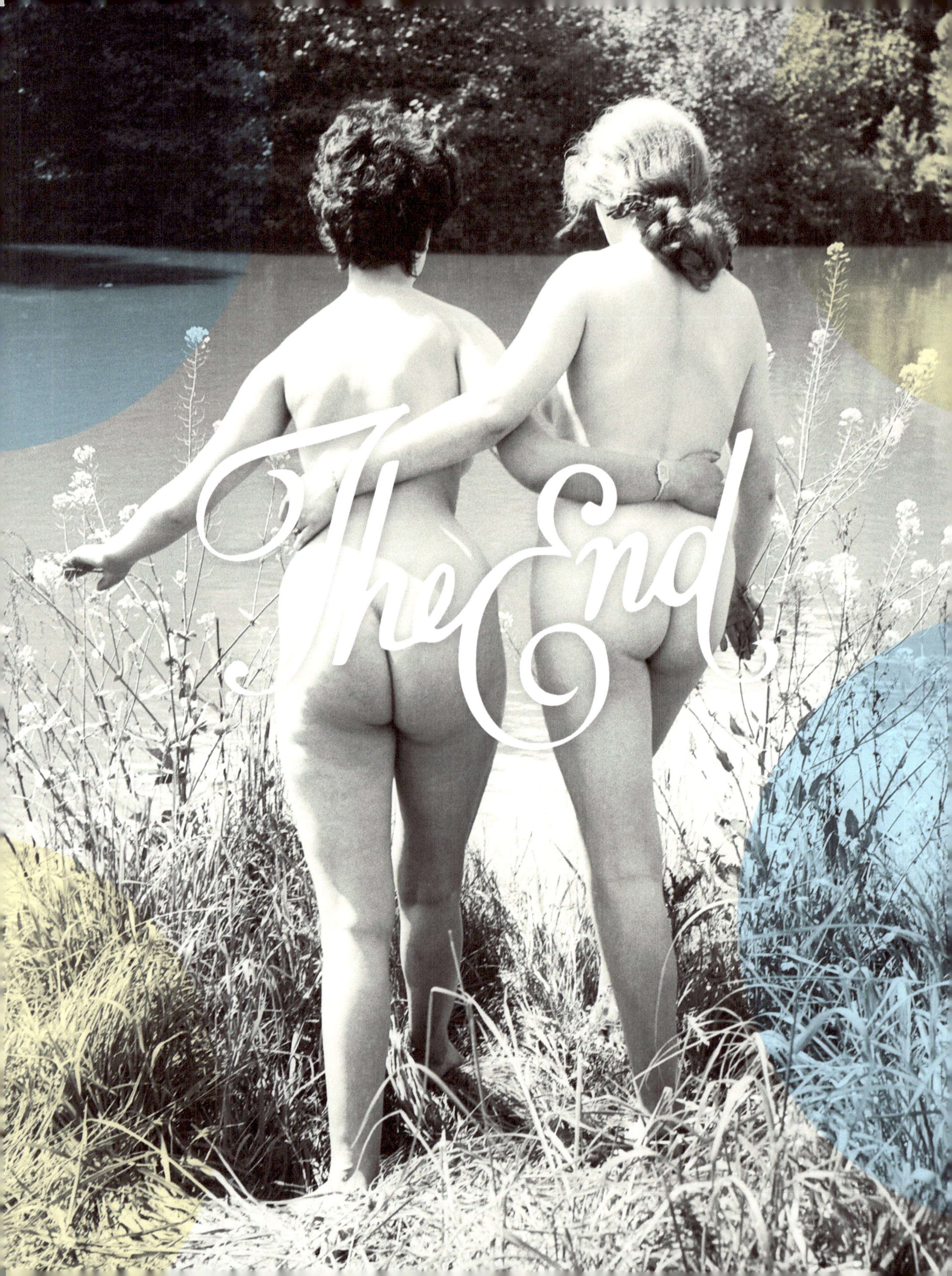
The End

www.ingramcontent.com/pod-product-compliance
Ingram Content Group UK Ltd.
Pitfield, Milton Keynes, MK11 3LW, UK
UKHW061034310726
14089UKWH00010B/235
9781916215160